Clinical Reasoning in Small An

Clinical Reasoning in Small Animal Practice

Jill E. Maddison

Director of Professional Development, Extra Mural Studies and General Practice
Department of Clinical Science and Services
The Royal Veterinary College

Holger A. Volk

Professor of Veterinary Neurology & Neurosurgery
Department of Clinical Science and Services
The Royal Veterinary College

David B. Church

Vice Principal for Learning and the Student Experience
The Royal Veterinary College

WILEY Blackwell

This edition first published 2015 © 2015 by John Wiley & Sons, Ltd

Registered office: John Wiley & Sons, Ltd, The Atrium, Southern Gate, Chichester, West Sussex, PO19 8SQ, UK

Editorial offices: 9600 Garsington Road, Oxford, OX4 2DQ, UK
The Atrium, Southern Gate, Chichester, West Sussex, PO19 8SQ, UK
1606 Golden Aspen Drive, Suites 103 and 104, Ames, Iowa 50010, USA

For details of our global editorial offices, for customer services and for information about how to apply for permission to reuse the copyright material in this book please see our website at www.wiley.com/wiley-blackwell

Library of Congress Cataloging-in-Publication Data

Maddison, Jill E., author.
Clinical reasoning in small animal practice/Jill E. Maddison, Holger A. Volk, David B. Church.
p. ; cm.
Includes bibliographical references and index.
ISBN 978-1-118-74175-7 (pbk.)
1. Veterinary medicine–Diagnosis. I. Volk, Holger A., author. II. Church, David B., author. III. Title.
[DNLM: 1. Animal Diseases–diagnosis. SF 771]
SF772.6.M33 2015
636.0896075–dc23

2014042409

A catalogue record for this book is available from the British Library.

Wiley also publishes its books in a variety of electronic formats. Some content that appears in print may not be available in electronic books.

Cover image: [Production Editor to insert]

Cover design by [Production Editor to insert]

Typeset in 11/14pt MeridienLTStd by Laserwords Private Limited, Chennai, India

1 2015

MIX
Paper from responsible sources
FSC® C013604

Contents

Contributors

Author affiliations

Dr. Jill E. Maddison BVSc, DipVetClinStud, PhD, FACVSc, MRCVS
Director of Professional Development, Extra Mural Studies and General Practice
Department of Clinical Science and Services
The Royal Veterinary College

Professor Holger A. Volk DVM, PGCAP, DipECVN, PhD, FHEA, MRCVS
Professor of Veterinary Neurology & Neurosurgery
Department of Clinical Science and Services
The Royal Veterinary College

Professor David B. Church BVSc, PhD, MACVSc, FHEA, MRCVS
Vice Principal for Learning and the Student Experience
The Royal Veterinary College

Foreword writer affiliations

Professor Stephen May MA, VetMB, PhD, DVR, DEO, FRCVS, DipECVS, FHEA
Deputy Principal
The Royal Veterinary College

Contributor affiliations

Mr Elvin R. Kulendra BVetMed, MVetMed, CertVDI, DipECVS, MRCVS
Lecturer in Small Animal Surgery
Department of Clinical Science and Services
The Royal Veterinary College

Dr. Andrea V. Volk Dr.med.vet, MVetMed, DipECVD, MRCVS
Staff Clinician in Veterinary Dermatology
Department of Clinical Science and Services
The Royal Veterinary College

Foreword

Although clinical reasoning and decision making are central to the veterinarian's (similar to the physician's) role, the process seems to be less well understood and associated with more erroneous statements about it in veterinary educational circles than any other of the skills we expect practitioners to possess. In an era that rightly prides itself on an evidence-based approach to medicine, it is surprising the way that increased repetition of statements such as 'students should not engage in pattern recognition', 'scientific method is used to reach diagnosis', 'analytical approaches are more accurate than pattern recognition' and 'at least with objective data you do not get biased interpretation' has led to them being accepted, even by those responsible for the education of the next generation of our profession.

In this book, Dr. Maddison and her colleagues aim to put the record straight through their clear description of their 'Logical Approach to Clinical Problem Solving' in the context of small animal practice. Their ideas have evolved from a combination of direct experience of the challenges of their different personal caseloads over many years and their reflections on how best to understand their expertise so that their methods could be explained to students in both the classroom and the clinic. However, with advances in our understanding of the way our brains work, we can increasingly link such insights to the approaches advocated in this book. We know that our processes of reasoning can be grouped into two categories (Evans 2003, 2012): type I (sometimes referred to as pattern recognition) and type II (analytical). Where possible in our lives, we try to use type I in making decisions, as it is rapid and efficient. It relies on our memory of similar problems encountered in the past, and, if we correctly apply such patterns, it is at least as accurate as analytical reasoning. However, our impulse for speed and efficiency, particularly in our busy modern world, can easily trap us into 'cognitive miserliness' (Stanovich 2009) where we do not take note of any lack of fit of our repertoire of patterns. In such circumstances, faced with 'high stakes' decisions such as the life and well-being of a patient, it is vital we cross-check our initial conclusions with an analytical approach, as this book emphasises (Ark *et al.* 2007).

Many continue to suggest that the analytical approach to clinical reasoning is 'scientific', involving hypothesis testing, but this is misleading. Scientific method involves us creating and testing hypotheses by predicting data and, subsequently, following an experiment, making observations on whether our predictions are correct. This has been called 'backwards reasoning'. It is extremely robust in the contexts in which it is relevant, but, particularly in primary care settings, where the number of possible diagnoses in an individual patient is large, such an approach quickly leads to cognitive overload. Even if a practitioner can persist in applying a hypothetico-deductive scientific approach, at this point, it is undermined by the very features that are meant to make it robust. The size of the potential data sets generated renders our decision making less accurate, and for novices, it can lead to 'paralysis by analysis', with a failure to act even when action is essential (Croskerry *et al.* 2014).

From observations of clinicians working with real and paper-based cases, clinical reasoning is an inductive process, working forward from data to diagnosis (Patel *et al.* 2005). This is the systematic approach adopted in this book, and it makes explicit for those starting to work with cases, and those who are more experienced, the intervening steps. In contrast to a backwards approach, which tends to fail to develop pattern recognition, this repeated use of systematic forward reasoning also helps to lay down structured patterns for future use (Sweller 1988). At an early stage, it is important to contain the size of the data set, and this is achieved by clustering signs to clarify the organ system (or systems) involved and how it is affected (Auclair 2007). Only then should we start to think about provisional diagnoses, and then this list will be much shorter than the series of lists, based on consideration of each clinical sign separately, that advocates of a 'scientific approach' have promoted in the past.

William Osler wrote that medicine is the *'practice of an art which consists largely in balancing possibilities (Osler 1910) .... It is a science of uncertainty and an art of probability ... Absolute diagnoses are unsafe and made at the expense of conscience'* (quoted in Bean 1968). His insight from 100 years ago reminds us that our diagnoses frequently remain provisional, in the sense that they are based on likelihood and may need to be modified as new information comes to light. Our approach is Bayesian, in the sense that these provisional diagnoses provide a prior probability in advance of further tests that we may undertake. Such tests can then be chosen on the basis that their result may increase the probability of our provisional diagnosis being correct. As a result of limitations of sensitivity and specificity, used in 'screening' mode, these tests can fail to detect many cases as well as yielding many false positive results. However, following a good clinical work-up and used in 'diagnostic mode', well-chosen tests can make us more confident in our diagnosis and plan to manage a case, still recognising that even with all the technology we possess, 'absolute diagnoses are made at the expense of conscience'.

Donald Schön, in his seminal work 'The Reflective Practitioner', uses two memorable images. He talks about specialist (academic) practice as occupying 'high, hard ground, overlooking a swamp' where it may be possible to solve problems with scientific approaches, and 'swampy lowland' where problems often appear messy and unclear, and where traditional scientific methods cannot apply (Schon 1983, p. 42). This book is meant for, and highly recommended to, all those who practice in the swamps! Another image Schön uses is of the expert pianist who tells a student that they need to modify their playing but cannot immediately say how (Schön 1995). The pianist has to sit at the piano and play the section to recognise the fingering that is required. The difficulty of the expert unpicking the detail of thinking processes that have become automatic, to teach them to others, is well known and can lead to misinterpretation, based on incorrect rationalisations of the processes involved. Therefore, this book is also highly recommended for all experienced practitioners keen to understand how their minds work, in order to support the learning of others in an evidence-based and proven way.

Stephen May

References

Ark, TK., Brooks, LR. and Eva, KW. The benefits of flexibility: the pedagogical value of instructions to adopt multifaceted diagnostic reasoning strategies. *Medical Education* **41**:281–287, 2007.

Auclair, F. Problem formulation by medical students: an observation study. *BMC Medical Education* **7**:16, 2007.

Bean WB. *Sir William Osler: aphorisms from his bedside teachings and writings.* 3rd ed Springfield, IL: Charles C Thomas; 1968, p 129.

Croskerry, P., Petrie, DA., Reilly, JB. and Tait, G. Deciding about fast and slow decisions. *Academic Medicine* **89**:197–200, 2014.

Evans, JStBT. In two minds: dual-process accounts of reasoning. *Trends in Cognitive Sciences* **7**:454–459, 2003.

Evans, JStBT. Spot the difference: Distinguishing between two kinds of processing. *Mind and Society* **11**:121–131, 2012.

Osler W. Teacher and Student. In *Aequanimitas, with other addresses to medical students, nurses and practitioners of medicine.* Philadelphia, PA: P Blakiston; 1910, p. 40.

Patel, VL., Aroche, JF. and Zhang, J. Thinking and reasoning in medicine, in K. Holyoak *Cambridge Handbook of Thinking and Reasoning.* Cambridge University Press, 2005. pp. 727–750.

Schon, DA. *The reflective practitioner: how professionals think in action.* San Francisco: Jossey-Bass; 1983.

Schon, DA. Knowing-in-action: the new scholarship requires a new epistemology. *Change: The Magazine of Higher Learning* **27**(6), 26–34, 1995.

Stanovich, KE. Rational and irrational thought: the thinking that IQ tests miss. *Scientific American Mind,* November/December, pp 34–39, 2009.

Sweller, J. Cognitive load during problem solving: effects on learning. *Cognitive Science* **12**:257–285, 1988.

Acknowledgement

We would like to thank our students, past and present, undergraduate and postgraduate, as well as practising veterinarians around the world who have worked with us. All have helped shape and inspire our teaching and learning around the concepts of clinical problem solving. We would also like to thank our colleagues Lucy McMahon, Ruth Serlin, Fran Taylor-Brown, Jane Tomlin and Martin Whiting for reviewing and providing insightful advice on early drafts of various chapters. And last, but by no means least, we are indebted to David Watson and Brian Farrow; without their insight, vision and inspiration, the wonderful journey this book represents would not have been possible.

CHAPTER 1

Introduction to problem-based inductive clinical reasoning

Jill E. Maddison & Holger A. Volk
The Royal Veterinary College, Department of Clinical Science and Services, London, UK

The aim of this book is to assist you to develop a structured and pathophysiologically sound approach to the diagnosis of common clinical problems in small animal practice. The development of a sound basis for clinical problem solving provides the veterinarian with the foundation and scaffold to allow them to potentially reach a diagnosis regardless of whether they have seen the disorder before. Furthermore, the method presented in this book will help you avoid being stuck trying to remember long differential lists and hence free your thinking skills to solve complex medical cases. The aim of the book is *not* to bombard you with details of different diseases – there are many excellent textbooks and other resources that can fulfil this need. What we want to provide you with is a framework by which you can solve clinical problems and place your veterinary knowledge into an appropriate problem-solving context.

We all remember our first driving lessons, which may have been quite challenging – for us and/or our instructors! We had to think actively about many factors to ensure we drove safely. The more experienced we became at driving, the more non-driving-associated tasks, such as talking to our passengers, listening to the radio and changing the radio channels, we were able to do while driving. If we had attempted any of these tasks at the beginning of our driver training, we might have had an accident. As we become more experienced at a task, we need to think less about it, as we move to what is known as unconscious competence.

Clinical Reasoning in Small Animal Practice, First Edition.
Jill E. Maddison, Holger A. Volk and David B. Church.

We see a similar process in clinical education. During the progression from veterinary student to experienced clinician, knowledge and skills are initially learnt in a conscious and structured way. Veterinary undergraduate education in most universities is therefore based on systems teaching, species teaching or a mixture of both. These are excellent approaches to help develop a thorough knowledge base and understanding of disease processes and treatments. However, when an animal or group of animals becomes unwell, the clinical signs they exhibit can be caused by a number of disorders of a range of different body systems – the list may seem endless. They do not present to the veterinarian with labels on their heads stating the disease they have (more's the pity!). Therefore, for the veterinarian to fully access their knowledge bank, they need to have a robust method of clinical reasoning they can rely on. This method allows them to consolidate and relate their knowledge to the clinical case and progress to a rational assessment of the likely differential diagnoses. This makes it easier to determine appropriate diagnostic and/or management options for the patient. Because you have a clear path, communication with the client becomes easier.

The next part of the journey of becoming an experienced clinician is that clinical judgement and decision-making processes become unconscious or intuitive. The rapid, unconscious process of clinical decision-making by experienced clinicians is referred to in medical literature as intuition or the 'art' of medicine. The conscious thinking process is often referred to as 'science' (evidence-based) or analytic. Intuition is context-sensitive, influenced by the level of the clinician's experience, context-dependent and has no obvious cause-and-effect logic. Why is this important? We have all thought – 'I just know that the animal has . . . .' The unconscious mind will pretend to the conscious mind that the clinical decision was based on logical assumptions or causal relationships. This is not a problem as long the intuition or 'pattern recognition' has resulted in a correct diagnosis. However, when it does not, we need to understand why it failed and have a system in place to rationally progress our clinical decision-making. This book will provide you with the tools and thinking framework needed to unravel any clinical riddle, unleashing the potential of your unconscious mind rather than blocking your working memory as you try to recall all the facts you may have once known.

Why are some cases frustrating instead of fun?

Reflect on a medical case that you have recently dealt with that frustrated you or seemed difficult to diagnose and manage. Can you identify why the case was difficult?

There can be a multitude of reasons why complex medical cases are frustrating instead of fun.

- Was it due to the client (e.g. having unreal expectations that you could fix the problem at no cost to themselves? Unwilling or unable to pay for the diagnostic tests needed to reach a diagnosis? Unable to give a coherent history?)
- Was the case complex and didn't seem to fit any recognisable pattern?
- Were you unable to recall all the facts about a disease and this biased your thinking?
- Did the signalment, especially breed and age, cloud your clinical decision-making resulting in an incorrect differential list?
- Did the case seem to fit a pattern but subsequent testing proved your initial diagnosis wrong?
- Did you seem to spend a lot of the client's money on tests that weren't particularly illuminating?

Can you add any other factors that have contributed to frustrations and difficulties you may have experienced with medical cases?

Apart from the client issues (and as discussed later, we may be able to help a little bit here as well), we hope that by the end of this book, we will have gone some way towards removing the common barriers to correct, quick and efficient diagnosis of medical cases and have made unravelling medical riddles fun.

Solving clinical cases

When a patient presents with one or more clinical problems, there are various methods we can use to solve the case and formulate a list of differential diagnoses. One method involves pattern recognition – looking at the pattern of clinical signs and trying to match that pattern to known diagnoses. This is also referred to as developing an illness script. Another method can involve relying on blood tests to tell us what is wrong with the patient – also referred to as the minimum database. Or we can use problem-based clinical reasoning. Often, we may use all three methods.

Pattern recognition

Pattern recognition involves trying to remember all diseases that fit the 'pattern' of clinical signs/pathological abnormalities that the animal presents with. This may be relatively simple (but can also lead to errors of omission) and works best:

- For common disorders with typical presentations
- If a disorder has a unique pattern of clinical signs
- When all clinical signs have been recognised and considered, and the differential list is not just based on one cardinal clinical sign and the signalment of the patient presented
- If there are only a few diagnostic possibilities that are
  - easily remembered or
  - can easily be ruled in or out by routine tests
- If the vet has extensive experience, is well read and up-to-date, reflects on all of the diagnoses they make regularly and critically and has an excellent memory.

Pattern recognition works well for many common disorders and has the advantage of being quick and cost effective, provided the diagnosis is correct. The vet looks good to the client because they have acted decisively and confidently ... provided the diagnosis is correct.

However, pattern recognition can be flawed and unsatisfactory when the clinician is inexperienced (and therefore has seen very few patterns) or only considers or recognises a small number of factors (and is not aware that this process is mainly driven by unconscious processes that might need to be reflected upon if they fail). Or even if the clinician is experienced, it can be flawed for uncommon diseases or common diseases presenting atypically, when the patient is exhibiting multiple clinical signs that are not immediately recognisable as a specific disease, or if the pattern of clinical signs is suggestive of certain disorders but not specific for them. In addition, for the experienced clinician, the success of pattern recognition relies on a correct diagnosis for the pattern observed previously being reached *and* not assuming that similar patterns must equal the same diagnosis. Pattern recognition can lead to dangerous tunnel vision where the clinician pursues his/her initial diagnostic hunch based on pattern spotting to the exclusion of other diagnostic possibilities. They may then interpret all subsequent data as favourable to their initial diagnosis, including ignoring data that doesn't 'fit' their preferred diagnosis. This phenomenon is described in psychological literature as confirmation bias – defined as a tendency for people to favour information that confirms their beliefs or hypotheses. And finally, the disadvantage of relying entirely on pattern recognition to solve clinical problems means that should the clinician realise subsequently that their pattern recognition was incorrect, they have no logical intellectual framework to help them reassess the patient. Thus, pattern-based assessment of clinical cases can result at best in a speedy, correct, 'good value' diagnosis but at worst in wasted time, money and, sometimes, endangers the life of the patient.

I'll do bloods!

Routine diagnostic tests such as haematology, biochemistry and urinalysis can be enormously useful in progressing the understanding of a patient's clinical condition. However, relying on blood tests (often called a minimum database) to give us more information about the patient before we form *any* assessment of possible diagnoses can be useful for disorders of some body systems but totally unhelpful for others. Serious, even life-threatening, disorders of the gut, brain, nerves, muscles, pancreas (in cats) and heart, for example, rarely cause significant changes in haematological and biochemical parameters that are measured on routine tests performed in practice. Over-reliance on blood tests to steer us in the right clinical direction can also be problematical when the results do not clearly confirm a diagnosis. The veterinarian can waste much time and the client's money searching without much direction for clues as to what is wrong with the patient. And of course, the financial implications of non-discriminatory blood testing can be considerable, and many clients are unable or unwilling to pay for comprehensive testing. Using blood testing to 'screen' for diagnoses can be misleading, as the sensitivity and specificity of any test are very much influenced by the prevalence of a disorder in the population.

For experienced veterinarians, pattern recognition combined with 'fishing expeditions' (i.e. 'I have no idea what's going on so I'll just do bloods and hopefully something will come up!') can result in a successful diagnostic or therapeutic outcome in many medical cases in first opinion practice. However, there are always cases that do not yield their secrets so readily using these approaches, and it is these cases that frustrate veterinarians, prolong animal suffering, impair communication, damage the trust relationship with clients and on the whole make veterinary practice less pleasant than it should be. You also have to know about *and* remember lots of diagnoses for this approach to be effective. This is problematical if the veterinarian does not recognise or remember potential diagnoses or if, as discussed previously, the pattern of clinical signs doesn't suggest a relatively limited number of differentials. It is also less useful for inexperienced veterinarians or veterinarians returning to practice after a career break or changing their area of practice.

It is for all of these reasons that we hope this book will enhance your problem-solving skills as well as build your knowledge base about key pathophysiological principles. We want to assist you to develop a framework for a structured approach to clinical problems that is easy to remember, robust and can be applied in principle to a wide range of clinical problems. The formal term for this is problem-based inductive clinical reasoning.

Problem-based inductive clinical reasoning

In problem-based inductive clinical reasoning, each significant clinicopathological problem is assessed in a structured way before being related to the other problems that the patient may present with. Using this approach, the pathophysiological basis and leading questions (see the following sections) for the most specific clinical signs the patient is exhibiting are considered before a pattern is sought. This ensures that one's mind remains more open to other diagnostic possibilities than what might appear to be initially the most obvious and thus helps prevent pattern-based tunnel vision. If there are multiple clinical signs, for example vomiting, polydipsia and a pulse deficit, each problem is considered separately and then in relation to the other problems to determine if there is a disorder (or disorders) that could explain all the clinical signs present. In this way, the clinician should be able to easily assess the potential differentials for each problem and then relate them rather than trying to remember every disease process that could cause that pattern of particular signs. It is important that the signalment of the patient is seen as a risk factor but should not blind the clinician to potential diagnoses beyond what is common for that age, breed and sex.

Thus, we *do* look for patterns but not until we have put in place an intellectual framework that helps prevent tunnel vision too early in the diagnostic process.

Essential components of problem-based clinical reasoning

Step 1 – the problem list

Construct a problem list

The initial step in logical clinical problem solving is to clarify and articulate the clinical problems the patient has presented with. This is best achieved by constructing a problem list – either in your head or in more complex cases, on paper or the computer.

Why is constructing a problem list helpful?

- It helps make the clinical signs explicit to our current level of understanding
- It transforms the vague to the more specific
- It helps the clinician determine which are the key clinical problems ('hard findings') and which are the 'background noise' ('soft findings')
- And most importantly, it helps prevent overlooking less obvious but nevertheless crucial clinical signs.

Identify the problems and 'prioritise'

Having identified the presenting problems, you then need to assign them some sort of priority on the basis of their specific nature.

For example, anorexia, depression and lethargy are all fairly non-specific clinical problems that do not suggest involvement of any particular body system and can be clinical signs associated with a vast number of disease processes. However, clinical signs such as vomiting, polydipsia/polyuria, seizures, jaundice, diarrhoea, pale mucous membranes, weakness, bleeding, coughing and dyspnoea are more specific clinical signs that give the clinician a 'diagnostic hook' they can use as a basis for the case assessment. As the clinician increases their understanding of the clinical status of the patient, the overall aim is to seek information that allows them to define each problem more specifically (i.e. narrow down the diagnostic options) until a specific diagnosis is finally arrived at.

Specificity is relative!

The relative specificity of a problem will, however, vary depending on the context. For example, for a dog that presents with intermittent vomiting and lethargy, vomiting is the most specific problem, as in all likelihood the cause or consequences of the vomiting will also explain the lethargy. In contrast, for the dog that presents with intermittent vomiting and lethargy *and* is found to be jaundiced on physical examination, jaundice is the most specific clinical problem. The majority of causes of jaundice can also cause vomiting but the reverse is not true, that is there are many causes of vomiting that do not cause jaundice. Thus, there is little value in assessing the vomiting as the 'diagnostic hook', as it will mean that many unlikely diagnoses are considered and time and diagnostic resources may be wasted. In this case, assessment of jaundice will lead more quickly to a diagnosis than that of vomiting, as the diagnostic options for jaundice are more limited than those for vomiting.

In other words, although you identify and consider each problem to a certain degree, you try to focus your diagnostic or therapeutic plans on the most specific problem (the 'diagnostic hook') if (and this is important) you are comfortable that the other clinical signs are most likely related. If you are not convinced that they are all related to a single diagnosis, then you need to keep your problems separate and assess them thoroughly as separate entities, which may or may not be related. There are reasons that might make one surmise that the clinical signs are related to more than one problem including the following:

1 The chronology of clinical signs is very different, raising the possibility that there is more than one disorder present.

2 The problems don't fit together easily, for example different body systems appear to be involved in an unrecognisable pattern.
3 Other clues that may be relevant to the case, for example some clinical signs resolved with symptomatic treatment but others didn't.

How do I decide what problems are specific?

As indicated previously, specificity is a relative term and will vary with each patient. There are a few clues that you can look for when trying to decide the most specific problems the animal has:

Is there a clearly defined diagnostic pathway for the problem with a limited number of systems or differential diagnoses that could be involved?

For example: vomiting vs. inappetance

- The problem of vomiting has a very clearly defined diagnostic pathway (discussed in Chapter 2), whereas there is almost an endless set of diagnostic possibilities for causes of inappetance, and there is no well-defined diagnostic approach (Chapter 4). Hence, vomiting is a more specific and appropriate 'diagnostic hook' than inappetance.

Could one problem be explained by all the other problems but not vice versa or does the differential diagnosis list for one problem include many diagnoses that would explain the other problems but not vice versa?

For example: vomiting vs. jaundice

- As mentioned earlier, jaundice is the more specific problem because most causes of jaundice could also conceivably cause vomiting, but there are many causes of vomiting that do not cause jaundice.
- Hence, the diagnostic pathway for jaundice is more clearly defined (discussed in Chapter 10), and there are a more limited number of possible diagnoses.

But don't forget to relate each problem to the whole animal

Once you have narrowed down your diagnostic options for the most specific problems, you use these to direct your diagnostic or therapeutic plans, but don't forget to consider the less specific problems in relation to your differential diagnosis.

For example, your *specific problem* may be polyuria/polydipsia (PU/PD) associated with a urine specific gravity of 1.002 (hyposthenuria), and your non-specific problem may be anorexia. Hence, when considering the potential differential diagnoses for PU/PD associated with hyposthenuria, those diagnoses for which anorexia is *not* usually a feature, for example psychogenic polydipsia, diabetes insipidus and hyperadrenocorticism, are much less likely than those diagnoses where anorexia is common such as hypercalcaemia, pyometra and liver disease. It is not always necessary to 'rule out' the former diagnoses, but they have a lower priority in your investigation than the latter group.

Thus, the thinking goes: '*the causes of hyposthenuria are ... ... (Chapter 12) and in this patient the most likely causes are ... ... (because of the other clinical signs or clinical pathology present).*" In other words, you use the non-specific problems to refine the assessment of the specific problems. One could claim that this is pattern recognition, and indeed it is to a certain extent. However, the step of clarifying the problem list (and thus not overlooking minor signs) and assessing the specific problems in this manner allows the clinician's mind to be receptive to differentials other than the supposedly blindingly obvious one that uncritical pattern recognition may suggest (such as thinking every cat with PU/PD must have renal failure). And as we discuss later in this chapter, the particular steps you take in assessing the specific problems also decrease the risk of pattern-based tunnel vision and confirmation bias.

How likely is a diagnosis?

Priority is also influenced by the relative likelihood of a diagnosis. Common things occur commonly. Therefore, although you shouldn't dismiss the possibility of an unusual diagnosis by any means, the *priority* for the assessment is usually to consider the most likely diagnoses first, provided they are consistent with the data available.

Step 2 – Does this make sense?

Always ask yourself, particularly when assessing clinical pathology or results of other diagnostic procedures in light of particular problems – '*does this make sense – does this clinicopathological abnormality explain the problem that the animal has?'* Good clinicians are good detectives!

Example 1

For example, a dog is depressed, anorectic, vomiting and polydipsic. Its blood glucose is 12 mmol/L (just above the reference range), it has 3+ glucosuria and no ketones in the urine. Does this mean that diabetes mellitus explains all of the dog's clinical signs? No – usually uncomplicated diabetes does not result in depression, anorexia and vomiting. There must be another reason for these clinical signs. Diabetic ketoacidosis might be occurring, but this has been ruled out by your urinalysis. Hence, you must look further for an explanation for the vomiting, anorexia and depression.

Example 2

Another example – an unwell dog (anorectic, vomiting and depressed) is found to have clinicopathological changes consistent with hyperadrenocorticism. Does this explain all of the dog's clinical signs? No – dogs with uncomplicated hyperadrenocorticism are not metabolically unwell, so there must be some other explanation for the dog's malaise that you will need to identify and resolve before definitive testing for hyperadrenocorticism is possible (because concurrent disease has a significant impact on dynamic adrenal testing).

Step 3 – think pathophysiologically

Another essential element is to think pathophysiologically. I'm sure that none of us realised when we were in vet school just how important an understanding of physiology and pathophysiology is to understanding medicine.

For example, an animal has profound hypokalaemia. Rather than trying to remember all the diseases that may cause hypokalaemia, review how the body might lose potassium or fail to acquire it or even 'use it up'. By getting into the habit of thinking in this manner, you can potentially diagnose disorders you may never have heard of (or that may never have been described before!). It will also stimulate you to seek more knowledge about the pathophysiology of disease processes, which will lead to a greater understanding of internal medicine and ultimately to a better retention of knowledge.

The problem-based approach

Problem-based approach means different things to different people, and you may have already read about or been to courses where it was discussed. Some regard the problem-based approach as meaning *'write a problem list, then list every differential possible for every problem.'* Not a feasible task unless you have an amazing factual memory and endless time! Others view the problem-based approach as meaning *'write a problem list, then list your differentials.'* This is really just a form of pattern recognition, but at least it makes a good start by formulating a problem list.

The basis of this book is the concept of problem-based inductive clinical reasoning, which is a more accurate definition than 'problem-based approach'. This approach provides steps to bridge the gap between the problem list and the list of differential diagnoses via a structured format. The problems should be investigated by rigorous use of the following questions:

- What is the problem?
- What system is involved and how is it involved?
- Where within the system is the problem located?
- What is the lesion?

The answers to these questions or the pursuit of the answers will determine the appropriate questions to ask in the history. They may alert you to pay particular attention to aspects of the physical examination. And/ or they may indicate the most appropriate diagnostic test to use to find the answers, as well as prepare you intellectually to assess the results of diagnostic procedures.

1 Define the problem

Example: the owner reports that the dog is vomiting. Is the animal really vomiting or regurgitating – or perhaps even coughing?

When considering the important clinical signs the patient is exhibiting, it is essential to try to define the problem as accurately as possible. *'A problem well defined is a problem half solved'* is a good maxim to work from. The first question to ask is *'is there another clinical sign that this problem could be confused with?'* This is a vital step, and failure to define the problem correctly has often derailed a clinical investigation that might otherwise have been relatively straightforward.

Other examples include the following:

- The owner says the dog is having fits – is it having seizures, episodes of syncope or vestibular attacks or other strange episodes? (Chapter 7)
- The owner says the dog has red urine – is it blood, haemoglobin or myoglobin? (Chapter 11).

1 Refine the problem

Some problems require further refining to clarify the best diagnostic approach.

Examples include the following:

- Weight loss – is this because of inappetance or despite a normal appetite? (Chapter 3)
- Collapse – with or without loss of consciousness? (Chapters 6 and 7).

Why is it so important to define and refine the problem?

The range of diagnoses to consider, diagnostic tools used and potential treatment or management options for clinical problems that may be perceived by the owner to be the same and present similarly to the veterinarian can be very different. Or the owner might perceive the presenting signs to be attributable to one problem, but in reality, the signs indicate another problem to the veterinarian. Failure to appropriately define and/or refine the problem can often lead to wasted time and money, as the wrong problem is investigated or treated. This can delay treatment, prolong the disease, prolong the patient's suffering, sometimes potentially endanger the life of the patient, may increase unnecessarily the costs to the client, frustrate the veterinarian *and* client and potentially impair the client–veterinarian relationship.

2 Define and refine the system

Once the problem is defined, the next step is usually to consider the system involved. For every clinical sign, there is a system(s) that *must* be involved, that is it 'creates' the clinical sign. However, the really important question is – how is it involved? The key questions in this case are *'what system is involved in causing this clinical sign?'* and *'do I have a primary i.e. structural problem of a body system or a secondary problem i.e. functional problem where the system involved is affected by other factors?'*

Examples include the following:

- The body system *always* involved when a patient vomits is the gastrointestinal (GI) system. However, it may be directly involved due to primary pathology of the gut such as parasites, inflammation, neoplasia and foreign body. This is defined as *primary (structural)* GI disease. Or vomiting may be occurring due to dysfunction of non-GI organs such as the liver, kidney, adrenal glands and/or pancreas. This is defined as *secondary (functional)* GI disease.
- The body system that is *always* involved when a patient has generalised weakness is the neuromuscular system. However, it may be directly involved due to *primary* neuromuscular pathology (e.g. inflammation, toxins, neoplasia and infection). Or the neuromuscular system may be malfunctioning due to the effect of pathology on other organs, causing metabolic derangements that impair neurological function such as hypoglycaemia, anaemia, hypoxia and electrolyte disturbances. This is defined as secondary neuromuscular disease.

Why is it so important to define and refine the system?

The range of diagnoses to consider, diagnostic tools used and potential treatment or management options for primary, structural problems of a body system are often very different compared to those relevant to secondary, functional problems of that system. Investigation of primary, structural problems often involves imaging the system in some manner (radiology, ultrasound, advanced trans-sectional imaging, endoscopy and surgery) and/or biopsy. Routine haematology, biochemistry and urinalysis are often of little diagnostic value. For secondary, functional disorders, on the other hand, haematology and biochemistry are often critically important in progressing our understanding of the case and reaching a diagnosis.

Failure to consider what body system is involved and how it is involved can often lead to wasted time and money. This can delay treatment, prolong the disease, prolong the patient's suffering, sometimes potentially endanger the life of the patient, may increase unnecessarily the costs to the client, frustrate the vet and client and potentially impair the relationship between vet and client. (Notice a recurring theme here?) In fact, if you do nothing else when assessing a case before seeking the diagnostic 'pattern', ask yourself for each of the specific problems – 'what system could be involved and how – primarily or secondarily?'. This simple question will immediately open your mind to diagnostic possibilities you may never have contemplated if you were just focusing on the 'pattern'.

Other examples include the following:

- Chronic cough – cardiac or respiratory system? (Chapter 8)
- Jaundice – due to prehepatic (haemolysis) or hepatic/post hepatic disorder? (Chapter 10)
- Cardiac arrhythmia – is it due to primary (structural) cardiac disease, for example dilated cardiomyopathy or extra-cardiac disease, for example gastric dilation and volvulus, splenic pathology? (Chapter 6)
- PU/PD – is it due to primary polydipsia or primary (structural) renal disease (chronic kidney disease) or extra-renal dysfunction, for example diabetes mellitus, hypercalcaemia and hypoadrenocorticism? (Chapter 12)

An alternative, although closely related, question for some problems is *'is the problem local or systemic?'*

- Epistaxis – due to local nasal disease or systemic disease, for example coagulopathy and hyperviscosity? (Chapter 11)
- Melaena – GI bleeding due to local disease (ulceration – which in turn may be due to primary or secondary GI disease) or systemic disease, for example coagulopathy? (Chapter 11)
- Seizures – due to local brain disease, for example neoplasia, infection/inflammation or systemic disease, for example electrolyte disturbances or intoxication (Chapter 7).

How to differentiate primary from secondary system involvement?

There are often clues from the history and/or clinical examination that help you define and refine the body system involved. Or you may not be able to answer this question until further diagnostic tests are performed. But just asking the question ensures that you remember that body systems can malfunction due to direct pathology of that system, for example inflammation, neoplasia, degeneration, infection or due to functional problems where factors not directly related to the body system can impact on its function.

3 Define the location

Example: having determined that vomiting is due to primary GI disease, where in the GI tract is the lesion located?

In this example, by asking this question, you will select the most appropriate method either to answer the question or to move on to the next step.

For example, if you believe that your history and physical examination and other ancillary data indicate a lower small intestinal lesion, endoscopy is not going to be an appropriate method of visualising the area or obtaining biopsies. However, if all the information you have suggests a gastric lesion, endoscopy may be most appropriate if available.

Other examples include the following:

- Vomiting due to secondary GI disease – liver, kidney, adrenals and pancreas? (Chapter 2)
- Hind limb weakness is due to neurological dysfunction – is the lesion in the spinal cord (and where), peripheral nerves, muscles or brain? (Chapter 6)
- Haematuria – from urethra, prostate, bladder or kidneys? (Chapter 11)

4 Define the lesion

Once the location of a problem within a body system is determined, usually the next key question is 'what is it?', that is you need to identify the pathology. It can be helpful to remember the types of pathology that can occur on broad terms – for example degeneration, anomaly, metabolic, neoplasia, nutritional, infection, inflammation, idiopathic ('genetic'), trauma, toxic and vascular (DAMNIT-V). Which type of pathology is most likely going to depend on the body system or organ involved, the signalment of the patient (species, breed, age, sex etc.), the clinical onset and course of the clinical signs, pain involvement, the geographic location of the patient and what disorders are common in that population.

This assessment can be influenced by whether the patient is in a general clinic or a referral hospital. Common things occur commonly or 'the hoof beats in the night are much more likely to be due to a horse than a zebra' (unless you are on safari of course!). This doesn't mean that uncommon diagnoses should not be considered (and they will of course be more common in referral hospitals). It's just that common disorders usually receive diagnostic priority at the beginning of a clinical investigation.

Example: the patient has a gastric lesion – is it a tumour, foreign body or ulcer?

This question will require visualisation and/or biopsy to answer, but it would have been a waste of time asking the question until you had arrived at the right location.

Other examples include the following:

- Spinal cord lesion visible on magnetic resonance imaging – is it inflammation, infection or a neoplasm?
- Haematuria is due to lower urinary tract disease – infection, calculi or neoplasia?
- Large bowel diarrhoea – parasites, infection, ulceration, stricture, neoplasia or diet related?

What do I need to do to define the problem, system, location or lesion?

The diagnostic methods used to define the problem, then the system, then, where appropriate, the anatomical location and then the lesion will vary depending on the problem.

For example, clinical pathology may be needed in some cases to define the problem, but in many cases, the problem will be definable on the basis of history (onset and course of the disease) and clinical examination findings. Similarly, diagnostic tests or procedures may be required to define and refine the body system involved in some cases, and for other problems, the system involved will be evident from clues from the history and/or the clinical examination. In some cases, once the problem is defined, for example regurgitation, the body system is immediately apparent and the anatomical location identified (upper GIT – oesophagus or pharynx). For neurological problems, clinical and neurological examination will often define the problem, system and location, leaving only the lesion needing to be defined by diagnostic testing.

Putting it all together

Defining the problem, system, location and then the lesion does not always follow this exact order. For some problems, for example coughing and diarrhoea, identifying the location occurs before identifying the system, as location identification helps identify the system (discussed in more detail in Chapters 3 and 8). For some problems, for example pruritus (Chapter 14), you might go straight from problem definition to seeking to define the lesion. However, for almost all clinical problems, answering *some or all* of the four questions – *'what is the problem? what system is involved and how? what is the location of the lesion? and what is the lesion?'* will provide a framework to guide your clinical reasoning and diagnostic and therapeutic decisions. Thus, instead of thinking when faced with a vomiting patient, 'I wonder if it has a gastric foreign body or renal failure or a liver tumour?', your initial energies are directed at defining the problem and system, which will help make your list of differentials (which are usually the location and/or lesion) logical, appropriate and given appropriate priority. In this way, the diagnosis is made thoughtfully, and during the process, all diagnostic options can be considered as the need arises.

But does pattern recognition have a place?

It is important to reiterate that pattern recognition for many cases is appropriate and justified – depending on your level of experience, knowledge, skill base and mindset. For example, if a pot-bellied elderly terrier with bilaterally symmetrical alopecia, seborrhoea, hyperpigmentation and comedones walked into your consulting room and the owner reported that the dog was drinking lots of water, was ravenously hungry and appeared to be panting excessively, then hyperadrenocorticism is the most obvious diagnosis, and going through the motions of assessing each specific problem would be ridiculous (but not if you had never seen a dog with hyperadrenocorticism before!).

However, it is important to be aware that pattern recognition is only foolproof if the pattern is virtually unique to the disease, you consider a sufficient number of factors in your pattern or there are a very limited number of diagnostic options. Its value is very dependent on the clinician's experience, depth of knowledge and ability to sort data quickly and efficiently.

Of course, once you have considered each individual problem, you do in fact look for a pattern in the clinical signs. However, the insertion of that initial step of considering each specific problem individually and *then* relating it to the other problems present should ensure that you don't miss the less obvious possible diagnoses.

In addition, the process of developing a sound problem-based approach can enhance your ability to pattern recognise because you have a greater understanding of the reasons *why* you believe certain patterns are suggestive of some disorders more than the others.

Combinations of clinical signs

There are some combinations/patterns of clinical signs that make the diagnostic options very limited, and it is entirely appropriate to consider them together; for example, the patient with PU/PD who is also polyphagic. If the PU/PD and polyphagia have been present for the same duration, then they are almost certainly due to the same disorder, and it is quite appropriate to assess them together. There are very few conditions that will cause this pattern of clinical signs (e.g. diabetes mellitus, hyperthyroidism and hyperadrenocorticism), so it is quite appropriate to concentrate on these first.

It may appear tedious at times!

You may feel at times that being asked to assess each individual's specific problem is a tedious exercise when the diagnosis is obvious, because you think you recognise the pattern of clinical signs. In some cases, this will be true, whereas in other cases, you will be misled. However, the most important point that we will try to get across is that if you don't 'practise' this structured problem-based approach on relatively simple clinical cases, when you are faced with the complex cases, which probably most of you feel frustrated about at present, you will not be able to apply problem-based principles and as such will be still left floundering as pattern recognition and/or going fishing fail you. It is also important to recognise that pattern recognition is a process of thinking that doesn't require explicit teaching – it happens naturally, whereas developing a robust structured inductive approach does require explicit articulation and practise of the steps involved.

Finding the right balance

It is also useful to remember that medical diagnoses are often based on the 'balance of probabilities' rather than having to be proved 'beyond reasonable doubt'. Striking the right balance between the diagnostic possibilities and judging what is important or likely and what is less important or less likely can be challenging and, of course, is very influenced by experience, but also understanding and knowledge.

Ancillary benefits

The aim of a structured and thorough approach to diagnosis is to reach the answer as quickly as possible and to get the best value from your 'diagnostic dollar/pathology pound/enabling euro' – that is not to waste the client's money on unnecessary tests and procedures. An additional advantage of following this approach is that you should have a very good idea *why* you are advising doing blood tests or taking radiographs or prescribing a particular medication. And because you know *why*, you can explain your reasons to the client clearly, and they are much more likely to agree to follow your suggestions. Client compliance is positively influenced by the degree to which they understand the reasons for diagnostic or treatment recommendations.

You are also in a much better position to explain the implications of 'normal results' rather than being sent into a panic because you were hoping the blood tests would show something ('because the dog looks really sick, so it must have an abnormal blood test! – but its blood results are absolutely normal! – HELP! – what do I do now?').

In conclusion

Problem-based inductive clinical reasoning:

- Is much more than just listing problem, then listing differentials for each problem (a common misconception about problem-based medicine).

- Has 'rules' that are easy to remember and can be applied to most clinical problems animals present with.
- Has a structured approach centred on three to four main steps as follows:
  - Define and refine the problem
  - Define and refine the system
  - Define the location (where appropriate)
  - Define the lesion
- Provides a framework to hang your knowledge on allowing you to recognise and retrieve more easily the information you need.
- Reduces the need to remember long list of differentials (see the first point).
- Helps prevent getting trapped by a perceived 'obvious' diagnosis – it helps avoid confirmation bias.
- Provides memory triggers to ensure an appropriate history is taken and a thorough clinical examination performed.
- Provides a clear rationale for choosing diagnostic tests or treatments that can be communicated to the owner.
- Helps turn a terrifying case into a manageable one!

Time waster or time saver?

It is common when first faced with the process of problem-based inductive clinical reasoning to feel that it is an academic exercise that there simply isn't time to apply in the context of a busy clinic, 10–15 min consultation slots and the many conflicting demands on your time. However, if you are able to put in the hard yards initially *and* if you discipline yourself to think in this manner, it will become second nature, subconscious (unconscious competence) and certainly not as laborious as it may appear at the beginning. In fact, acquisition of these problem-solving skills will ultimately save time, as it will help you quickly eliminate extraneous background noise and focus on what is important for the patient and client. An analogy is the process of learning a new language. To do so, you initially need to learn some vocabulary and grammar (framework), but once you have a basic understanding *and* if you use the new language on a daily basis, further progression to fluency comes naturally. But without the basic framework and constant practice, fluency is an unfulfilled dream.

Comments from participants in courses based on this approach include that they developed 'a more systemic approach to medicine, which *saved a lot of time* in a busy practice'; 'it made me *think more efficiently* in a busy practice'. Hopefully, this will be your experience too. As with all skills, it takes time to develop the knowledge base and mental discipline required for this form of clinical reasoning, but once developed, it will provide a firm base for the future and, most importantly, will not 'go out of date', no matter how many new diseases/disorders are discovered.

CHAPTER 2

Vomiting and regurgitation

Jill E. Maddison
The Royal Veterinary College, Department of Clinical Science and Services, London, UK

Vomiting is a very common clinical sign in small animal practice. The main function of vomiting is to protect the animal from ingested toxins. Dogs in particular have a propensity to eating disgusting things and have a very well-developed vomiting reflex. The causes and consequences of vomiting can range from clinically inconsequential to life threatening. In contrast, regurgitation is a much less common clinical sign. Almost invariably, the patient who is truly regurgitating will have serious disease. It is therefore essential that the clinician has a robust and rapid way to assess patients during the initial consultation so that rational decisions can be made about appropriate diagnostic and/or therapeutic plans.

Physiology

In order to develop a rational approach to the patient who is reported to be vomiting, it is important to appreciate the pathophysiology of vomiting and regurgitation.

Vomiting or emesis is the forceful expulsion of gastric contents through the oesophagus, mouth and, sometimes, nostrils. It is a neurologically complex process resulting from the synchronised activity of a number of abdominal, pharyngeal and thoracic structures. The act of vomiting is coordinated in the medulla oblongata and cannot occur without a functional vomiting centre. In contrast, regurgitation is a passive process, which involves the retrograde movement of food and fluid from the oesophagus, pharynx and oral cavity without the initiation of reflex neural pathways other than the gag reflex.

Clinical Reasoning in Small Animal Practice, First Edition.
Jill E. Maddison, Holger A. Volk and David B. Church.

The essential neurological components of the emetic reflex are the following:

- Visceral receptors
- Vagal and sympathetic afferent neurones
- Chemoreceptor trigger zone (CRTZ)
- Vomiting centre within the reticular formation of the medulla oblongata.

It is important to understand the stages that occur in the act of vomition, as they contribute to the clinical manifestation of vomiting, and this also assists the clinician to differentiate vomiting from regurgitation.

The first stage of vomiting is *nausea*. In this stage, gastric tone is reduced, duodenal and proximal jejunal tone is increased and duodenal contents reflux into the stomach. The patient often appears depressed, hypersalivates and as a result may exhibit repeated swallowing and/or lip licking behaviour.

The nauseous stage is followed by *retching* (an unproductive effort to vomit, also known as 'dry heaves') and then *vomiting*. When the animal vomits, the epiglottis is closed and the soft palate presses up against the nasopharynx. The abdominal muscles and the diaphragm contract. The contraction of the abdominal muscles is usually visible to an observant owner. The cardia then opens, the pyloric stomach contracts and vomiting occurs. Reverse peristalsis, cardiac rhythm disturbances and increased colonic motility also occur during the vomiting process.

The closure of the epiglottis and pressing of the soft palate up against the nasopharynx protect against aspiration of gastric contents. In contrast, during regurgitation, which is a passive process without neurological coordination, these actions do not occur. As a result, aspiration pneumonia is a common sequela to disorders which cause regurgitation and less likely in vomiting unless the animal is obtund.

Initiation of and the process of vomiting

Vomiting is essentially initiated by either humoral or neural pathways. The *humoral pathway* involves stimulation of the CRTZ within the medulla oblongata by blood-borne substances; the *neural pathway* is through activation of the vomiting centre.

Vomiting centre

All animal species that vomit have a brainstem 'vomiting centre', which is a group of several nuclei that act in concert to coordinate the somatomotor events involved in expelling gastric contents. Non-vomiting species such as horses, rodents and rabbits also have the brainstem nuclei and motor systems necessary for emesis but lack the complex synaptic interaction between the nuclei and viscera required for a coordinated reflex.

There does not appear to be a discrete vomiting centre within the reticular formation of the medulla oblongata. Rather, there is an 'emetic complex' that refers to groups of loosely organised neurons distributed throughout the medulla, which are sequentially activated and play a role in emesis. This complex will be referred to in this chapter as the vomiting centre, however, as conceptually this assists the understanding of the physiology and pathophysiology involved.

The vomiting centre receives input from vagal and sympathetic neurones, the CRTZ, the vestibular apparatus and the cerebral cortex. It may also be stimulated directly by blood-borne toxins that can cross the blood brain barrier (BBB).

Central stimulation

Central stimulation of the vomiting centre occurs via higher centres in the central nervous system (CNS). Stimuli include nervousness, unpleasant odours, pain and psychogenic factors. Opioids and benzodiazepine receptors have been implicated in centrally initiated vomiting, but their exact mode of action has not been well characterised pharmacologically. Centrally induced vomiting may also occur due to direct stimulation of the emetic centre by elevated cerebrospinal fluid pressure, encephalitis or CNS neoplasia.

Vestibular apparatus

Labyrinthine dysfunction associated with motion sickness and middle/inner ear infection also has input into the vomiting centre via neural pathways arising from the vestibular system. The CRTZ is involved in this pathway in the dog but not the cat.

Chemoreceptor trigger zone

The CRTZ is located in the area postrema in the floor of the 4th ventricle. It has no BBB, therefore allowing toxins and chemicals that would normally be excluded from the CNS access to the brain. The CRTZ is stimulated by endogenous toxic substances produced in acute infectious diseases or metabolic disorders such as uraemia or diabetic ketoacidosis, as well as by drugs and exogenous toxins.

Peripheral receptors

Peripheral receptors are located mainly in the gastrointestinal (GI) tract, particularly the duodenum, but also in the biliary tract, peritoneum and urinary organs. The receptors may be stimulated by distension, irritation, inflammation or changes in osmolarity. There are a few receptors in the lower bowel, which explains why patients with inflammatory lower bowel disease may occasionally vomit.

Assessment of the patient reported to be vomiting

1 Define the problem

It is very important to differentiate vomiting from regurgitation. It is also important to differentiate the vomiting animal from one that has a productive cough and gags after coughing. This is often confused with vomiting by owners. Owners are often unable to differentiate between vomiting, regurgitating and gagging. It is important to ask specific questions (and perhaps even find ways to illustrate the differences such as acting out retching movements or abdominal effort) to elicit appropriate information, for example amount of effort involved, character of vomitus and so on. If still uncertain, the veterinarian may need to observe the animal and/or proceed with diagnostics appropriate to both regurgitation and vomiting.

Why is it important to differentiate vomiting from regurgitation?

The differential diagnoses, appropriate diagnostic tools and management strategies are completely different for patients who are vomiting compared to those who are regurgitating, gagging or coughing (caused by respiratory or cardiac disease).

Patients who are vomiting (due to primary GI or secondary GI disease) may be treated symptomatically or investigated, depending on the case, using a variety of diagnostic tools, including clinical pathology, diagnostic imaging, endoscopy and exploratory laparotomy.

When regurgitation is the predominant clinical sign, it will usually be due to oesophageal disease (very occasionally pharyngeal) and usually carries a poor or guarded prognosis due to the type of lesion – for example foreign body, stricture or megaoesophagus. The patient should not be treated symptomatically without diagnostic investigation to define the lesion where possible. In addition, the investigation of regurgitation essentially involves visualising the oesophagus (by endoscopy and/or diagnostic imaging tools) – it is rare for routine clinical pathology to be of diagnostic value in defining the type of lesion (megaoesophagus, foreign body etc.), although it may be of value once megaoesophagus is diagnosed in assessing the possible causes.

Similarly, the patient who is gagging most likely has a lesion in the pharyngeal region or upper oesophagus, and visualising the lesion is the appropriate diagnostic path. Clearly, the animal that is coughing has respiratory or cardiac disease and requires an entirely different diagnostic approach.

Failure to define the problem appropriately can therefore potentially endanger the patient and may lead to wasted time and money and impair the veterinarian–client relationship and trust.

Clues to help differentiation of vomiting, regurgitation, coughing and gagging

Patients who vomit behave differently compared to those who regurgitate. As discussed, vomiting is a neurologically coordinated activity with defined stages and physical manifestations. The patient will exhibit abdominal effort before bringing up the material, and vomiting is often preceded by hypersalivation – manifested by licking of lips and repeated swallowing (which are signs of nausea). The vomiting may be projectile. In contrast, regurgitation is a passive process – there are no coordinated movements. It is often induced or exacerbated by alterations in food consistency and exercise and facilitated by gravity when the head and neck are held down and extended. Animals that regurgitate will often gag as the material accumulates in the pharynx.

The character of the material expelled may also give the clinician clues. While undigested food may be brought up by vomiting or regurgitation, if the food is partially digested and/or contains bile, the patient is vomiting and not regurgitating. The pH of the vomitus is occasionally, but not always, useful. Acidic material strongly suggests vomiting, but pH neutral material may be the product of either vomiting or regurgitation.

As mentioned, because the epiglottis does not close, regurgitating patients are at considerable risk of aspirating gastric contents. Thus, if an owner reports that his/her animal developed a cough at the same time it starts 'vomiting', the clinician should be alert to the possibility that aspiration has occurred and that this is more likely to occur with regurgitation than vomiting.

There is a caveat, however, which should be kept in mind. Patients who have experienced serious vomiting of acidotic gastric contents may develop a secondary oesophagitis and present with signs suggestive of both vomiting *and* regurgitation. Usually, vomiting will have been the first sign noted. Animals that ingest caustic or irritant material causing oesophagitis and gastritis may also present with signs of both vomiting and regurgitation.

2 Define and refine the system

Primary vs. secondary gastrointestinal disorders

Reviewing the physiology of vomiting as discussed in the previous section and as shown in Figure 2.1, it is apparent that vomiting may occur due to primary GI disease or from secondary or non-GI disease.

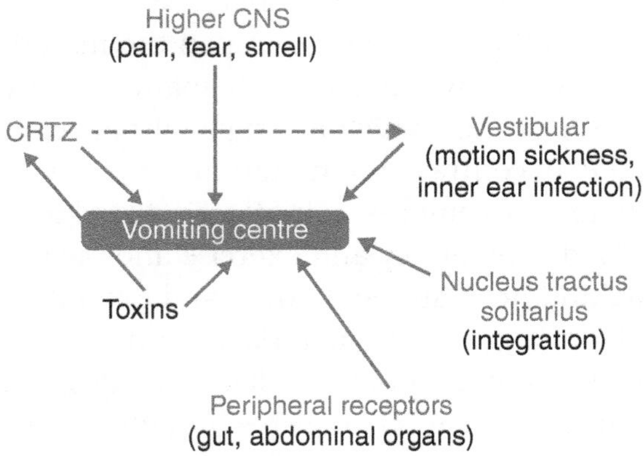

Figure 2.1 The relationship between the elements of the emetic reflex.

Table 2.1 Oesphageal disorders causing regurgitation.

Megaoesophagus	• Congenital	
	• Acquired – primary GI	• Idiopathic
	• Acquired – secondary GI	• Polymyositis • Myasthenia gravis • Polyneuritis • Hypothyroidism • Hypoadrenocorticism • Neoplastic neuromyopathy • Lead toxicity • Tick paralysis (*Ioxodes holycyclus*)
External compression	• Persistent right aortic arch • Mediastinal lymphoma • Thyroid tumours	
Internal obstruction – physical or functional	• Foreign body • Oesophagitis • Stricture	
Intramural Lesions	• Neoplasm • Abscess • Granuloma	

In contrast, regurgitation is almost always due to primary oesophageal disease (Table 2.1).

Primary GI diseases are those where there is specific primary GI pathology such as gut disturbance due to dietary indiscretion, inflammation, infection, parasites, obstruction or neoplasia. There may be metabolic consequences of the GI disease, but the *primary pathology is in the GI tract*.

Secondary GI disease is where the vomiting or regurgitation has occurred due to *pathology elsewhere in the body* – the gut is just the 'messenger'. Abnormalities of other body systems may indirectly cause vomiting either due to the action of toxins on the CRTZ, vomiting centre and vestibular system or by stimulation of peripheral non-GI-associated vomiting receptors. Examples would include renal failure, liver disease, ketoacidososis, pancreatitis, hypercalcaemia, hypoadrenocorticism and other metabolic disorders. In most cases, there is no pathology identifiable in the gut, or where there is, for example ulceration secondary to liver or renal disease or hypoadrenocorticism, the primary cause is the metabolic disorder. While symptomatic management strategies might be directed at the gut pathology in these cases (such as the use of anti-ulcer drugs), there is no diagnostic benefit to imaging the gut, for example by endoscopy.

Why is it important to differentiate primary from secondary GI disease?

It is important to determine whether primary or secondary GI disease is occurring in the vomiting or regurgitating animal, as much time and money can be wasted if the wrong system is investigated. As discussed in Chapter 1, the range of diagnoses to consider, diagnostic tools used and potential treatment or management options for primary, structural problems of a body system such as the GI tract are often very different compared to those relevant to secondary, functional problems of that system. Investigation of primary GI disease often involves some form of imaging modality (radiology, ultrasound, endoscopy and surgery) and/or biopsy. Routine haematology and biochemistry are often of little diagnostic value in GI disease, although they may give clues about the clinical status of the patient. In contrast, for secondary GI disorders, haematology, biochemistry and other tests are often critically important in progressing towards a diagnosis.

It is also important to appreciate that there are cases of primary GI disease causing vomiting such as gastroenteritis caused by ingestion of spoiled food or other irritants that can be safely treated symptomatically, as the cause is transient and will resolve within days without specific treatment. Symptomatic management such as withholding food, antiemetic treatment and/or dietary change is appropriate for these patients. However, there are few, if any, secondary GI causes of vomiting (such as liver disease, renal failure, hypoadrenocorticism and hypercalcaemia) where the cause is transient, which will respond to symptomatic treatment and/or will resolve without specific therapeutic intervention.

The uncommon secondary GI causes of regurgitation all cause megaesophagus (Table 2.1), so the clinical decision pathway leading to their diagnosis begins with the diagnosis of megaoesphagus by endoscopy or diagnostic imaging and *then* the search for a metabolic cause. As mentioned, symptomatic treatment of regurgitation without establishing the cause is not prudent.

Thus, the clinician's clinical reasoning, *in the consultation room,* about whether primary or secondary GI disease is likely to be present is a crucial component of the rational management of patients reported to be vomiting or regurgitating and of clear communication with the client.

What are the clues that the patient has primary or secondary GI disease causing vomiting?

Primary GI disease should be strongly suspected if:

- an abnormality is palpable in the gut, for example foreign body and intussusception;
- the vomiting is associated with significant diarrhoea;
- the patient is clinically and historically normal in all other respects;
- the onset of vomiting significantly preceded any development of signs of malaise – depression and/or anorexia;
- the vomiting is consistently related in time to eating (although this can also occur with pancreatitis).

It is important to note, however, that primary GI disease cannot be ruled out even if none of the aforementioned features is present. For example, vomiting may be delayed for some hours (up to 24 h) in animals with non-inflammatory gastric disorders. Animals with foreign bodies or secretory disorders of the bowel often vomit despite not eating. In lower bowel disorders, vomiting more commonly occurs at variable times after eating.

Animals with primary GI may also be depressed and inappetant due to the lesion (there are neural inputs to the satiety centre in the hypothalamus from the gut) or due to the secondary effects of prolonged vomiting such dehydration or electrolyte disturbances. Usually, the malaise will occur at the same time or after the onset of vomiting.

Thus, the features in the aforementioned bulleted list are strong clues that primary GI disease is present, but their absence does not preclude it.

Animals with secondary GI disease are vomiting due to the effect of toxins on the vomiting centre or CRTZ or because of the stimulation of non-GI-associated peripheral receptors. The vomiting is usually unrelated to eating – *except pancreatitis in dogs*.

Animals with secondary GI disease will:

- Often have evidence from the history and/or clinical examination of abnormalities affecting other organ systems, for example jaundice, polydipsia/polyuria.
- Vomiting is usually intermittent, unrelated to eating and may often occur subsequent to the onset of other signs of malaise.
- In general, animals that are vomiting due to extra-GI disease are metabolically ill and are not usually bright, alert and happy.
- If a patient has been metabolically ill (depressed and inappetant) for a significant period *before* vomiting was observed, then secondary GI disease is most likely.

Secondary GI causes of regurgitation will frequently have other systemic signs such as generalised weakness or metabolic malaise. It is usually only patients with megaoesophagus due to focal myasthenia gravis who present with regurgitation as their only clinical sign.

Exceptions to the 'rules'

The exception to these generalisations about the features of secondary GI disease is pancreatitis in dogs. Canine pancreatitis behaves similar to a primary GI disease – it causes acute-onset vomiting in an initially often otherwise well dog; the vomiting often occurs immediately after eating, and decreased appetite and depression may not precede the onset of vomiting. Pancreatitis in cats, however, usually behaves similar to a secondary GI disease. Cats with hyperthyroidism may also vomit intermittently over a prolonged period and seem otherwise well (although, of course, they may also have other clinical signs suggestive of hyperthyroidism).

3 Define the location

If primary GI disease is determined to be present, the temporal relationship of vomiting to eating and the character of the vomitus should be used to assess where the lesion is likely to be – the upper or lower GI tract.

Diagnostic tools such as contrast radiography may be appropriate to localise the lesion. An assessment of the likely location of the lesion is important, as this may determine what further diagnostic procedures are suitable. For example, endoscopy would be appropriate for examining the stomach and possibly duodenum but will be of little use if lower small bowel disease is suspected.

Defining the location for secondary GI disease usually involves routine clinical pathology, dynamic or function tests +/− imaging to localise the organ affected, for example liver, kidney, pancreas and adrenals.

The location of the problem for patients who are regurgitating is always the oesophagus, whether the cause is primary or secondary GI. Thus, regurgitation is a clinical sign where location is considered first and then the question is asked – is this a primary or secondary GI lesion?

4 Define the lesion

Primary GI diseases causing vomiting

Once the lesion has been located within the GI tract, it must now be identified. Biopsy may be appropriate or the type of lesion may be evident by visual inspection (e.g. foreign body).

In the GI tract, as elsewhere, neoplasia and inflammation often look grossly identical, and biopsies should always be taken. Even if the GI tract looks grossly normal, biopsies should be obtained.

Diseases of the stomach

- Gastritis
  - dietary indiscretion
  - drug induced
  - immune mediated
  - eosinophilic
  - infection, for example *Helicobacter pylori*
- Gastric foreign bodies
- Gastric ulceration
  - *Note that gastric ulceration can be due to either primary GI lesion, for example secondary to a foreign body, inflammatory disease or neoplasia but can also be caused by secondary GI disease such as mastocytoma, liver disease, uraemia, pancreatic neoplasia (gastrinoma) and drugs such as NSAIDs.*

- Disorders of the pylorus
  - Pylorospasm
  - Pyloric obstruction
  - Congenital pyloric stenosis
  - Chronic hypertrophic gastropathy
- Abnormal gastric motility

Intestinal disease

Those intestinal diseases for which vomiting is a predominate clinical feature include the following:

- Enteritis, for example parvovirus, corona virus and dietary indiscretion
- Intestinal obstruction – foreign body and intussusception
- Inflammatory bowel disease especially in cats (dogs tend to more commonly present with diarrhoea as the major clinical sign).

The closer the obstruction is to the pylorus, the more frequent and severe the vomiting.

Secondary GI diseases causing vomiting

A large number of secondary GI disorders can cause vomiting. However, most of these can be eliminated with relatively few tests – at least in dogs. Cats are more problematical especially in the diagnosis of pancreatic and hepatic disease. In Table 2.2, the most important secondary GI disorders are listed with tests that are useful in their diagnosis.

You should consult other textbooks to read about specific details of primary and secondary GI diseases causing vomiting and regurgitation.

Diagnostic approach to the patient reported to be vomiting

It is imperative to carefully evaluate the history and physical examination findings for any clues that indicate whether the patient is vomiting or regurgitating and may suggest secondary or primary GI disease. You cannot always determine from the history and physical examination whether primary or secondary GI disease is most likely, but it is important that you ask yourself the questions: – ***I****s this patient vomiting or regurgitating? and* ***D****oes this patient have primary or secondary*

Table 2.2 Secondary gastrointestinal causes of vomiting in cats and dogs.

Disorder	Useful clinical pathology
Pancreatitis	Pancreatic lipase immunoreactivity (PLI), amylase (not in cats), lipase (not in cats), white blood cell count (WBC) count, ALP
Hepatic disease	ALT, ALP, GGT, bile acids, bilirubin
Renal disease	Urea, creatinine, phosphate, urine specific gravity (SG)
Hypoadrenocorticism	Na^+, K^+, urea, cortisol
Diabetic ketoacidosis	Blood and urine glucose, ketones
Toxaemia due to infection	WBC count
Hypercalcaemia	Serum Ca^{2+} (total and ionised)
Hypokalaemia/ hyperkalaemia	Serum K^+
CNS disease	Cerebrospinal fluid (CSF) analysis (possibly)
Dirofilariasis (cats)	Heartworm antigen tests (often negative), eosinophil count
Lead toxicity	Blood lead and/or urinary delta-aminolevulinic acid (δ-ALA)
Hyperthyroidism (cats)	Thyroxine (T4) (vomiting is intermittent and not severe)

GI disease or I can't tell?, as this will assist in directing your history taking and physical examination as you search for clues to enable you to answer these key questions.

In some vomiting cases, it will be obvious that primary GI disease is most probable (e.g. the bright, happy dog that, for several days, has been vomiting consistently half an hour after eating and has no other systemic signs). Or it may be clear that secondary GI disease is most likely (e.g. the cat that has been intermittently vomiting for a week, inappetant for 4 weeks and is also polydipsic). However, often, you cannot be sure based on the history and physical, so your diagnostic procedures will be aimed initially at answering the question 'What system and how?' You won't always be able to answer the question, but it is essential that you ask it.

If indicated by the history and/or physical examination, investigate secondary GI disease with appropriate diagnostic tools such as biochemistry, haematology and urinalysis. Only a proportion of vomiting animals will require a diagnostic work-up, but it is still important to consider whether primary or secondary GI disease is likely, as this will influence your symptomatic treatment.

As discussed earlier, the most common causes of primary GI disease, such as gastritis due to dietary indiscretion, will usually respond satisfactorily to symptomatic treatment (which should rarely, if ever, include antibacterial treatment). However, most secondary GI disease will not, and further information is required for management and prognosis.

When is clinical pathology useful?

In general, clinical pathology is most useful for progressing our understanding about secondary GI diseases causing vomiting. In contrast, for most primary GI disease, clinical pathology tests may provide information about the systemic effects of vomiting but *not* about the aetiology of the gut disorder.

Even if primary GI disease is strongly suspected, it may be helpful to perform appropriate tests to assess the patient's hydration and electrolyte/acid–base status, as prolonged and severe vomiting may cause biochemical derangements such as alkalosis or acidosis, prerenal azotaemia, hypokalaemia, hyponatraemia and hypochloraemia. Noting, however, that diagnostic procedures aimed at visualising the GI tract such as plain and/or contrast or endoscopy are more diagnostically useful in primary GI disease. Ultrasonography or exploratory laparotomy can be useful diagnostically for both primary or secondary GI disorders.

If you are unable to determine from the history and physical examination whether the animal has primary or secondary GI disease, it is cheaper, less invasive and usually quicker to investigate secondary GI disease first with appropriate tests and *then* investigate primary GI disease as needed if clinical pathology is normal. If there is any risk that patient has an intestinal obstruction, then plain abdominal radiographs should be performed as soon as possible. And if the patient has a concurrent cough, then this requires urgent investigation, as a serious disorder causing regurgitation is very possible.

When is a fuller work-up rather than symptomatic therapy indicated?

In general practice we obviously do not investigate every vomiting patient presented to us. Symptomatic treatment is quite appropriate if an assessment has been made by the clinician that the patient is vomiting, not regurgitating and probably has primary GI disease of a transient nature such as dietary indiscretion or food intolerance. A fuller work-up involving clinical pathology (either for diagnostic information or to assess the systemic effects of vomiting) +/– imaging is indicated if:

- the patient is regurgitating
- there has been no response to symptomatic therapy
- vomiting is persistent and severe
- other systemic signs are present, such as PU/PD and icterus
- inappetance and/or depression that commenced well before the onset of vomiting
- the patient is severely depressed
- there is a palpable abnormality in the gut.

In conclusion

Veterinarians in general practice frequently assess animals whose owners report they are vomiting. A structured clinical approach based on the key questions of defining the problem/system/location/lesion provides a robust framework for the clinician, which ensures that all relevant clues are considered. Seeking the answers to the key questions should be the driving force behind diagnostic and therapeutic decision making. The thinking skills, once acquired, allow a rapid assessment in the consultation room of these key questions, provide a firm foundation for clinical decision making and immeasurably assist in client communication.

CHAPTER 3
Diarrhoea

Jill E. Maddison
The Royal Veterinary College, Department of Clinical Science and Services, London, UK

Diarrhoea is a common clinical sign in animals presented to veterinarians in small animal practice. Similar to vomiting, the clinical consequences can range from insignificant to life threatening, although the latter is less common than the former. Many acute cases require little diagnostic intervention and resolve with or without symptomatic treatment. Chronic diarrhoea, however, can be a diagnostic challenge and the source of much frustration for the client and veterinarian. Animals can have chronic diarrhoea for months to years. Often, the animal may not be particularly unwell, the diarrhoea may be chronic but intermittent and may respond partially but not entirely to different therapeutic interventions.

Diagnostic investigation of chronic diarrhoea can involve various procedures that range from the inexpensive to the expensive and the non-invasive to the invasive – unfortunately, often with no middle ground between the extremes. Unlike many clinical problems, therapeutic trials often play an important role in helping the clinician reach a probable diagnosis. However, trials need to be conducted logically and the outcomes reviewed critically. The temptation to give multiple treatments aimed at different aetiologies in the hope that something will work is understandable. But even if there is a positive response to multi-modal therapy, if the diarrhoea recurs once treatment stops (as it often does), the clinician is no wiser about the underlying cause and how to manage the patient long term. Patience is needed by all parties, and excellent communication between the veterinarian and the client is imperative. As such, the clinician needs to have a clear diagnostic approach and a good understanding of the pathophysiology of diarrhoea and its causes. A rational diagnostic and therapeutic

Clinical Reasoning in Small Animal Practice, First Edition.
Jill E. Maddison, Holger A. Volk and David B. Church.

approach to chronic diarrhoea in the dog and cat is dependent on a basic understanding of the function of the gut and the classification of the type of diarrhoea that is present.

Classification of diarrhoea

Although symptomatic therapy is appropriate for the majority of animals with acute diarrhoea, chronic diarrhoea usually does not respond to non-specific symptomatic treatment and will often present the veterinarian with a diagnostic challenge where the more routine laboratory aids are not useful.

The diagnostic work-up, differential diagnoses and therapy for small and large bowel diarrhoea may differ, although there are some common causes. Therefore, it is of utmost importance that, before embarking on invasive diagnostic procedures or extensive therapy, an assessment is made as to whether the diarrhoea is:

- Acute or chronic
- Relatively mild or more severe with the presence of secondary systemic effects
- Small bowel or large bowel origin, or mixed
- Due to primary or secondary GI disease.

Failure to elicit sufficient information from the client about the characteristics of the diarrhoea, so as to allow appropriate classification as small bowel, large bowel or mixed, may result in inappropriate diagnostic procedures with increased expense to the client and frustration of the veterinarian, client and patient.

1 Define the problem

Diarrhoea is defined as an alteration in the normal pattern of defaecation, resulting in the passage of soft, unformed stools with increased faecal water content and/or increased frequency of defecation. It is important to consider the animal's previous pattern of defecation, as the frequency of defaecation and the nature of faeces vary between individuals.

There are a few uncommon situations where it may not be obvious to the owner that their animal has diarrhoea. Occasionally, they may mistake anal or vaginal discharges for diarrhoea, or see vomitus on the floor and think it is diarrhoea. The patient with constipation may pass small amounts of liquid faeces, which the owner thinks is diarrhoea. Conversely, the patient who is straining to defaecate and attempting to defaecate frequently as a result of large bowel disease may be interpreted by the owner as being constipated. Therefore, it is important that the clinician is cognisant of these issues and aims to define the problem as a first priority in the consultation.

Define the location

In cases of diarrhoea, the problem-based system we discussed in Chapter 1 is applied, but in a slightly different order. Identification of the *location* occurs first, which *then* assists in defining the *system*. This is because almost always, large bowel diarrhoea reflects primary GI disease, whereas small bowel diarrhoea can occur with either primary or secondary GI disease. Thus, defining the location *first* aids in defining the system.

A thorough history is essential to differentiate small from large bowel disease. It is important to carefully question the owner as to the character of the faeces and to elicit information regarding consistency, colour, frequency and presence of blood or mucus. Related abnormalities should also be assessed, such as whether there has been significant weight loss, loss of appetite or vomiting. The characteristics of small and large bowel diarrhoea are detailed in Table 3.1.

Because large bowel diarrhoea has fewer and more specific characteristics than small bowel diarrhoea, it is often easiest to note if there is any fresh blood, mucous and small amounts of faeces passed frequently. If the diarrhoea has none of these characteristics, then the patient has small bowel diarrhoea. Note also that diarrhoea may have features of *both* small and large bowel, which indicates either primary small bowel with secondary effects on the lower bowel or diffuse disease involving both the small and large intestine.

Define the system

Diarrhoea can be due to primary disorders of the small bowel and/or large bowel or to other systemic, secondary GI disorders such as

Table 3.1 Characteristics of small and large bowel diarrhoea.

	Small bowel diarrhoea	Large bowel diarrhoea
Consistency, amount and pattern	• Faecal bulk and/or water content is increased. Diarrhoea may be projectile and does not usually involve significant tenesmus.	• Small amounts of faecal material are passed frequently. Tenesmus is often present, particularly if the lower colon or the rectum is involved.
Blood	• If blood is present, it is usually digested (melaena) or in acute diarrhoea, reddish-brown.	• If blood is present, it will be undigested (haematochezia).
Appearance	• Colour may be grey if large amounts of undigested fat are present or if the diarrhoea is due to lactose intolerance. A yellow-green coloration is common and due to malabsorbed bile salts.	• Mucus is often present either on the surface (indicating the lesion is in the lower colon or rectum) or throughout the faeces (indicating a lesion in the higher colon).
Weight loss	• Chronic small bowel diarrhoea is often (but not always) associated with weight loss.	• Usually there is no weight loss.
Vomiting	• Vomiting may also be present (but need not be). Relationship to eating can be variable depending on the location of the lesion.	• Vomiting can occur especially but is infrequent and is unrelated to eating.

Borborygmus and flatulence	• Gas commonly occurs with small bowel diarrhoea, as malabsorbed carbohydrates are fermented by colonic bacteria producing CO_2 and H_2S.	
Appetite	• Appetite may be variable depending on the underlying aetiology.	• Usually, the appetite is unaffected.
Water balance	• If the diarrhoea is severe, the animal may be dehydrated. If the diarrhoea is very watery, the patient may have an increased water intake.	• Large bowel diarrhoea *per se* does not usually adversely affect water balance.
Physical examination	• Physical examination may reveal increased gas or thickened loops of bowel but is often unrewarding. Always do a rectal examination to check for melaena or large bowel signs such as mucus and fresh blood about which the owner may not be aware of.	• Physical examination is often unremarkable, but it is imperative to do a rectal examination to check for strictures, masses or thickened mucosa.

hepatic disease, pancreatic insufficiency, pancreatitis, hyperthyroidism or hypoadrenocorticism. As discussed earlier, large bowel diarrhoea is almost always due to primary GI disease, whereas small bowel diarrhoea may occur with either primary or secondary GI disease. Severe systemic toxicity and uraemia can cause large bowel diarrhoea, but this will be a very minor clinical sign in relation to the patient's other clinical signs. Thus, it does not really pose a realistic diagnostic option when considering the work-up of a patient whose primary problem is large bowel diarrhoea.

Diarrhoea due to primary GI disease is more common than diarrhoea due to secondary GI disease. In animals with secondary GI disease, with the exception of pancreatic insufficiency, diarrhoea is *not* usually the primary presenting complaint.

4 Define the lesion

The following tables summarise the causes of acute and chronic small and large bowel diarrhoea (Tables 3.2–3.4).

Diagnostic approach to the patient with diarrhoea

Small bowel diarrhoea

Acute vs. chronic

It is important to ascertain the duration the diarrhoea has been present. Acute diarrhoea that is not severe, fulminating and potentially life threatening does not usually require extensive diagnostic investigation and will usually respond to non-specific therapy. Fulminating acute diarrhoea (e.g. viral and haemorrhagic gastroenteritis [HGE]) may not require extensive diagnostic testing but will require intense supportive therapy and should not be treated on an outpatient basis if at all possible. In contrast, chronic diarrhoea persisting for weeks to months indicates that a more thorough investigation is required.

When to investigate?

If the diarrhoea persists despite symptomatic treatment or is chronic, severe and associated with significant weight loss and/or evidence

Table 3.2 Causes of acute small bowel diarrhoea in dogs and cats.

Cause	Examples	Comments
Diet related	• Overeating (especially pups) • Dietary change • Spoiled food • Dietary indiscretion	Including change to food that causes allergy/hypersensitivity.
Parasites/protozoa	• Parasites ∘ most commonly ascarids (*Toxocara* and *Toxascaris* spp., also hookworms *Ancylostoma* and *Uncinaria* spp.) • Protozoa ∘ *Giardia* spp. ∘ Coccidia, for example *Cystoisospora* spp. (formerly called *Isospora*) ∘ *Cryptosporidium* spp.	Direct examination of fresh faeces for *Giardia* trophozoites may be useful, although a positive result may be coincidental as *Giardia* sp. can be found in the faeces of dogs without diarrhoea. Direct examination for *Giardia* spp. is not very sensitive, and thus many false negatives will occur, especially if only one faecal sample is examined. Zinc sulphate flotation is a sensitive test, provided three faecal samples are examined (~95% sensitive). A negative result does not necessarily exclude Giardia infection, and some clinicians will treat with metronidazole or fenbendazole regardless and proceed with further investigations only if the diarrhoea persists. The ELISA test can identify Giardia antigen in faeces. The test is reported to be about 90% sensitive and is probably more sensitive than performing a single zinc sulphate flotation examination.

(*continued overleaf*)

Table 3.2 (*continued*)

Cause	Examples	Comments

Infection (bacterial/viral)	• Viral enteritis
	  ◦ parvo
	  ◦ corona
	  ◦ distemper
	  ◦ other viruses (e.g. adenovirus, norovirus?)
	• bacterial enteritis
	  ◦ *Campylobacter* spp.
	  ◦ *Salmonella* spp.
	  ◦ *E. coli*
	  ◦ *Clostridium* spp.
		Microbial culture of faeces is often unrewarding due to the abundant normal flora in the gut and the predominance of anaerobes. *E. coli* is frequently, and *Salmonella* sometimes, isolated from faeces of normal animals, and therefore their presence does not necessarily imply that they are the cause of the diarrhoea. *Campylobacter* spp. and *Clostridium* spp. are also found in both animals with and without diarrhoea, which makes interpretation of results quite difficult.
		On a practical level, consider faecal culture when diarrhoea is acute and haemorrhagic, very severe, or in multiple animals in a crowded environment such as a kennel environment. If the owner or the pet is immunocompromised or if the owner is also affected with diarrhoea, this may also be a good time to consider faecal culture. Overall, most dogs and cats with diarrhoea do not required faecal culture; it rarely adds to the clinical picture, and it increases the overall cost of investigation.
		Clostridium perfringens and *Clostridium difficile* have equal prevalence in dogs with and without diarrhoea. However, there is a correlation between the presence of diarrhoea and the detection of toxins that are produced by these bacteria. Identification of an overgrowth of Clostridia or Clostridial spores on faecal smears means nothing diagnostically and will occur in many situations when gut flora is disturbed by a variety of GI disorders.

Toxins	• Toxins ∘ lead ∘ organophosphates ∘ plants	Plants that may cause diarrhoea if ingested (as well as other clinical signs) include Lily of the Valley, daffodil bulbs, Aloe vera, asparagus fern, chrysanthemums and cyclamens.
Unknown	• Haemorrhagic gastroenteritis (HGE)	HGE is a syndrome causing acute onset of vomiting and bloody diarrhoea. Characteristically, the patient will have significant haemoconcentration (increased PCV) with a normal or low plasma protein due to protein loss in the bowel. It usually occurs in small breed dogs. The cause is unknown – it is postulated that it may be due to hypersensitivity or a result of toxin production by *Clostridia perfringens*.
Secondary GI disease	• Acute pancreatitis severe systemic disease	See previous comments regarding presence of other clinical signs.

Table 3.3 Causes of chronic small bowel diarrhoea in dogs and cats.

Cause	Examples	Comments
Diet related	• Diet-responsive disease or food responsive enteropathy	Food intolerance is a non-immunological reaction to a component of food, for example gluten, preservative, bony material and other irritants. Food allergy/hypersensitivity is an immunological reaction to a component of food, for example beef and dairy. Diagnosis of dietary allergy or intolerance is usually a process of trial and error by using elimination diets, as there is no sensitive or specific diagnostic test. True dietary hypersensitivity may or may not be associated with peripheral eosinophilia (i.e. hypersensitivity should not be ruled out if the eosinophil count is normal). Current evidence would suggest that blood tests for anti-food antibodies are not specific and not clinically useful.
Parasites/protozoa	• Intestinal parasites (as previously mentioned) • Protozoa (as previously mentioned)	See comment in Table 3.2.
'Infection'/ bacterial/viral	• *Campylobacter/Salmonella* • FIP	Note comments in Table 3.2 in relation to bacterial causes of diarrhoea.
Antibiotic responsive	• Idiopathic antibiotic responsive diarrhoea (ARD) • Secondary SIBO	ARD: small intestinal diarrhoea that is responsive to antibacterials but no underlying cause can be identified. SIBO: small intestinal bacterial overgrowth secondary to an underlying problem such as exocrine pancreatic insufficiency, inflammatory bowel disease, partial obstruction or motility disorders.

Infiltrative	• Inflammatory bowel disease (IBD) • Diffuse lymphosarcoma • Adenocarcinoma • Mast cell tumour (feline)	Diarrhoea is the most common clinical signs of IBD in dogs. Vomiting is the more common clinical sign in cats. Intestinal biopsy is primarily required to characterise infiltrative inflammatory gut disease (IBD vs. neoplasia) and/or protein-losing enteropathy. Intestinal biopsy is indicated if small intestinal disease is confirmed by appropriate means, and factors such as parasites, bacterial (including ARD) or dietary causes are ruled out.
Miscellaneous	• Lymphangiectasia • Brush border enzyme biochemical defects • Selective cobalamin deficiency	Lymphangiectasia is usually secondary to IBD.

Secondary GI	• Motility disorders, for example
	  ∘ hyperthyroidism
	  ∘ lead toxicity
	  ∘ dysautonomia
	• Hypoadrenocorticism
	• Exocrine pancreatic insufficiency
	• Hepatobiliary disease
	• Severe systemic disease	

Table 3.4 Causes of acute and chronic large bowel diarrhoea in dogs and cats.

Parasites/protozoa	• *Trichuris vulpis* (whipworm) • *Ancylostoma caninum* (hookworm) • *Giardia* spp. (more commonly small bowel but can affect both) • *Tritrichomonas foetus* (cats) • *Entamoeba* spp.
Infection (bacterial/viral)	• *Campylobacter* spp. • *Clostridium perfringens; Clostridium difficile.* • *Salmonella* sp. • *Yersinia enterocolitica* • FIP
Diet related	• Diet-responsive disease (dietary allergy or dietary intolerance) • Passing foreign material • Fibre deficient diet

Inflammatory	• Inflammatory bowel disease
	  ◦ lymphocytic-plasmacytic enteritis (colitis)
	  ◦ eosinophilic enteritis (colitis)
	• Histiocytic colitis (Boxer dogs)
	• Granulomatous colitis

Neoplasia	• Diffuse or focal lymphosarcoma • Adenocarcinoma/adenoma • Mast cell tumour (feline) • Smooth muscle/stromal cell tumours (canine)
Stress	• Stress-induced colitis can occur relatively commonly in hospitalised dogs. This may reflect overgrowth of *Clostridium* spp.
Strictures	• Scar or neoplastic (adenocarcinoma)

of hypoproteinaemia, dehydration or systemic illness, then a more detailed investigation is indicated. Only a small proportion of diarrhoea cases requires investigation as chronic disorders. An animal presenting with intermittent but repetitive episodes of diarrhoea over many months should also be considered for investigation unless there is a proven cause (e.g. regular garbage bin raiding).

The following is an outline of a pragmatic approach to the patient with diarrhoea seen in general practice.

1. If the diarrhoea is acute, if appropriate for the patient, advise fasting for up to 24 h or feed small, more frequent meals of a bland, low residue diet (chicken/cottage cheese/rice or appropriate commercial product).
2. Ensure the worming history is up-to-date, and if in doubt, treat with a broad spectrum anthelmintic. Consider using fenbendazole as the first choice, as it is effective against helminthes and *Giardia*. If large-bowel diarrhoea is present, do a faecal flotation if possible. If *Trichuris vulpis* is present, the patient will need to be wormed at two-monthly intervals indefinitely, as the environment will remain contaminated due to the robust nature of the eggs.
3. Perform a direct saline smear wherever possible to check for protozoa such as *Giardia* and *Tritrichomonas foetus*.
4. If there has been no response to fasting and/or fenbendazole treatment, then consider treatment with metronidazole (10–20 mg/kg bid) before any expensive, invasive or time-consuming investigations are initiated.
5. At this point the vast majority of cases have resolved. However …
6. Ensure that secondary GI disease is not present, for example hyperthyroidism, hepatic disease and hypoadrenocorticism.
   (a) Even if the electrolytes are normal, if the patient does *not* have a stress leukogram, consider doing an adrenocorticotropin (ACTH) stimulation test to rule out hypoadrenocorticism before any invasive tests, for example biopsy.
7. Assuming that you are comfortable that the patient has primary GI disease, if small bowel diarrhoea persists after points 1–4 for more than a week or so (depending on the severity, the animal's clinical condition and owner concerns), consider treating for

antibiotic responsive diarrhoea (ARD) with oxytetracycline, tylosin or amoxicillin.

- Four to six weeks of therapy is usually the recommended treatment. The most appropriate drug has not been determined by controlled clinical trials.
- Occasionally, these patients respond to increased fibre diets (commercial or adding unprocessed bran).
- The role of probiotics in cases of idiopathic ARD has yet to be determined, but anecdotal reports suggest such therapy is unrewarding. This may be related to the fact that appropriate (e.g. host species specific) agents have yet to be used.

8 If the patient still has diarrhoea, consider a faecal culture for *Campylobacter, Salmonella* and *Escherichia coli,* and if available, request tests for Clostridial toxins (but note that false positives are possible) and/or assess for *Tritrichomonas* in a cat (may do this earlier in the process if pure bred or from a multi-cat household or shelter).

9 And/or (depends on the severity of the diarrhoea, client factors such as finances etc.) recommend commencement of a diet trial (commercial or home made, novel protein source or hydrolysed). Discussion with the owner will include the fact that dietary hypersensitivity is worth checking for as (a) the next step will be gut biopsy and (b) dietary change is the first management decision when inflammatory bowel disease (IBD) is detected by biopsy. Diet will be recommended for 4–6 weeks, but if there is absolutely no response after 2 weeks, then the prognosis for a good response is reduced.

10 And/or (if the owner will not/cannot comply with the dietary trial and/or the patient has large bowel diarrhoea but with not a lot of fresh blood – just mucus and tenesmus) advise adding fibre to the diet (unprocessed bran or soluble).

- It is probably prudent *not* to combine a hypoallergenic diet with fibre addition, because if the patient responds, you don't know which component they have responded to – the diet or the fibre – which has significant implications for future dietary recommendations (not to mention the wallet of the client).

11 If all the above mentioned fails *or* if the patient is hypoproteinaemic *or* if the patient has really bloody large bowel diarrhoea and severe tenesmus *or* if there is any other clue that neoplasia may be the cause, ideally advise ultrasound (by a specialist) and/or biopsy – either by endoscopy, if equipment and expertise are available, or by exploratory laparotomy.

Factors to consider in relation to decision making about biopsies

It is often not wise to biopsy an animal with chronic small or large bowel diarrhoea that is otherwise well and has no clues that there may be infiltrative disease (e.g. serious weight loss, hypoproteinaemia, palpable gut abnormality and ultrasound evidence of gut pathology) until it has been:

- Wormed
- Treated with metronidazole
- Considered for an antibacterial trial for ARD
  - Tetracycline
  - Tylosin
- Undergone a proper dietary trial – hypoallergenic and fibre

Why?

If biopsy confirms IBD, this is not a single disease, and detection of GI inflammation does not necessarily confirm IBD that requires immunosuppressive therapy. A proportion of patients with IBD will respond to antibiotics (they may have dysbiosis – abnormal gut flora population and/or abnormal response to normal flora) or dietary change. Of those who don't, it is believed that they may have a genetic immune defect. Some of these animals will respond to immunosuppressive treatment, but for a small group unfortunately, no treatment is effective.

Thus the key questions to be answered by biopsy are as follows:

- Does this patient have IBD, which will require treatment with immunosuppressive drugs?
- Does this patient have neoplasia?
- Does this patient have primary or secondary lymphangiectasia?

In conclusion

Veterinarians frequently assess animals with diarrhoea in general veterinary practice. Many cases will be transient and respond to symptomatic management. Those cases that are chronic can be a source of great frustration for all concerned. A structured approach to their assessment by ensuring that the type of diarrhoea is classified and using a judicious mix of diagnostic tests and therapeutic trials to define the lesion can greatly improve therapeutic outcomes.

CHAPTER 4
Weight loss

Jill E. Maddison
The Royal Veterinary College, Department of Clinical Science and Services, London, UK

Weight loss or failure to gain weight is a relatively common problem in small animal practice. The weight loss may be noticed by the owner or may be detected by the veterinarian or nurse when comparing weight records from previous visits to the veterinary hospital. Weight loss may be clinically inconsequential, for example moderate weight loss associated with a pet's increased activity in the summer months, or an indication of disease. Depending on other clinical signs, it may be a non-specific problem, which will be explained when the more specific problems are assessed. Or it may be the 'diagnostic hook' that forms the core of the clinician's clinical assessment and reasoning.

1 Define the problem

The first step when an animal is presented for weight loss is to *ensure that the caloric intake and palatability of the diet are adequate* for the animal's needs. Owners of large and giant breed dogs particularly may inadvertently underestimate the dog's caloric requirement, especially if the dog is growing or is very active. The normal caloric requirement of a normally active dog or cat can be calculated using the following formula:

$$[(30 \times \text{weight in kg}) + 70] \times 1.2\ \text{kcal}$$

This can probably be doubled for a growing dog, a very active animal or one that is pregnant or lactating. As a rough guideline, one cup of standard dry food is approximately 400 kcals and 400 g, wet food approximately 360 kcals. Only if the diet and caloric intake

Clinical Reasoning in Small Animal Practice, First Edition.
Jill E. Maddison, Holger A. Volk and David B. Church.

are adequate for the animal's life stage and style can weight loss be regarded as a manifestation of disease.

It can sometimes be difficult to distinguish general weight loss from severe muscle wasting causing loss of body weight and the appearance of emaciation. Therefore, while all of the following diagnostic approaches are appropriate for loss of body weight with a normal or increased appetite, keep in mind that very occasionally one may be dealing with muscle atrophy for which the system involved (neuromuscular – see Chapters 6 and 7) and type of disorders (infectious, immune mediated etc.) are very different.

Refine the problem

A crucial step in assessing the patient who has lost weight is to consider the weight loss in the context of the animal's appetite. Weight loss conditions are divided into the following:

- Those associated with a decreased appetite
- Those where the appetite is normal or increased.

Weight loss due to decreased appetite

Can't eat or won't eat?

If the owner reports that an animal is not eating, the first key question is 'is it because the animal can't eat or won't eat?' It is important to ensure that the animal does not have any condition causing difficulties in prehension or mastication or a swallowing defect – dysphagia ('can't eat').

True loss of appetite ('won't eat') may occur in many disease conditions. Loss of appetite is a frequent presenting complaint, as owners will usually be aware of the amount of food eaten by their pet, and it is often the first indication to an owner that there is something wrong.

Appetite is controlled by feeding-satiety centres of the hypothalamus, and many factors will directly or indirectly influence this centre, for example blood glucose levels, body temperature, metabolic products, electrolyte balance, blood calcium levels, neural input from the gastrointestinal tract, substances released by neoplasia and neurobehavioural factors (e.g. stress and fear). Particularly in cats, loss of the sense of smell may cause anorexia, and hence nasal disorders may need to be investigated.

Can't eat

Abnormalities of prehension, mastication or swallowing

Prehension and mastication

The animal with prehension or mastication difficulties can appear hungry and interested in food. They are either unable to pick food up properly, show evidence of pain when trying to eat or drop food from their mouth when chewing. Prehension and mastication difficulties are most often associated with disorders of the mouth and pharynx.

Local disorders of the mouth include the following:

- inflammation
- ulceration
- foreign bodies
- dental disease
- neoplasms.

Less commonly, impaired prehension or mastication may be due to inflammation of the muscles of mastication (myositis) or neuromuscular lesions resulting in paralysis of the muscles of the jaw or tongue. The muscles of mastication innervated by cranial nerve V (trigeminal), and the tongue by cranial nerve XII (hypoglossal).

Dysphagia

Difficulty in swallowing (dysphagia) is indicated by excessive, forceful attempts to swallow or by regurgitation of food from the mouth or nostrils.

Dysphagia can be due to the following:

- Local disorders of the tongue or pharynx such as inflammation, foreign bodies, trauma or neoplasia.
- Palatine abnormalities
- Rarely, neurological disorders involving cranial nerve IX (glossopharyngeal), cranial nerve X (vagus) or cranial nerve XII (hypoglossal) may be responsible.
- Cricopharyngeal achlasia is a rare congenital disorder of young animals in which the cricopharyngeal sphincter fails to relax when the animal swallows. Its aetiology is unknown, but it is surgically correctable by a cricopharyngeal myotomy.

Assessment of inflammation

Inflammation of the lips, gums, tongue, gingival or oropharyngeal structures may cause problems with prehension, mastication or swallowing. Inflammation can be due to local disease or systemic disease.

Systemic disorders include the following:

- Uraemia due to renal failure
- Viral infections in cats (tongue)
- Autoimmune disorders (pemphigus)
- Neutropenia
  - drug dyscrasias, for example phenylbutazone and phenobarbitone
  - bone marrow failure, for example FeLV associated

Local disorders include the following:

- Irritants (plant and chemical)
- Foreign bodies (often wedged across the hard palate)
- Dental disease
- Eosinophilic complex of cats
- Lymphocytic/plasmacytic stomatitis.
- Neoplasms
  - Benign
    - Papillomas
    - Epulis
  - Malignant – unfortunately, the majority of oral tumours are malignant. The most common ones are the following:
    - malignant melanoma
    - squamous cell carcinoma
    - fibrosarcoma

Won't eat

Anorexia/inappetance

When an animal is presented because of anorexia or inappetance with no other clinical abnormalities, in many cases, a thorough physical examination will reveal more specific abnormalities that can be investigated, for example pyrexia, masses, severe constipation, severe heart disease, anaemia and icterus.

However, in some cases, an underlying cause cannot be found on physical examination alone. In these cases, the diagnostic approach is partly dependent on the duration the animal has been anorectic and the degree of weight loss that has been sustained.

For an animal that has not eaten for 24–48 h and is in good bodily condition with no evidence of malaise, it may be most appropriate to adopt a 'wait and see' approach – to advise the owner that if the cause of the loss of appetite is serious, the animal is most likely to develop other clinical signs such as vomiting or diarrhoea that may help localise the problem. It is important in these cases to determine whether the diet has been changed recently or whether there are environmental conditions that may be responsible, for example very hot weather, absent owner, new pet or baby in the house and change of ownership or house.

If the anorexia is prolonged and/or the animal has lost significant weight and/or is exhibiting signs of non-specific malaise, then further diagnostic procedures are indicated. As a plethora of disease processes can cause anorexia, for example liver disease, renal failure, neoplasia, infection, electrolyte imbalance, endocrine abnormalities, anaemia and toxins, it can appear a daunting task to determine the cause.

2 Define the system

Diagnostic procedures should be directed at trying to determine the system involved and should, if possible, start with non-invasive or more cost-efficient tests and then proceed to more invasive or more expensive procedures if indicated.

Appropriate tests to evaluate inflammation/infection, serum protein, liver and renal function, electrolytes and calcium levels should be performed. In cats, viral infections such as FeLV and, more commonly, FIP should be considered. In appropriate geographic areas (where lead toxicity is recognised to occur), lead toxicity should be considered, as cats with lead toxicity may present with anorexia as their only clinical sign. In an older animal, a more rigorous search for neoplasia (e.g. abdominal and thoracic imaging) may be indicated.

Weight loss with normal or increased appetite

Weight loss syndromes associated with a normal or increased appetite can be divided into the following:

- *Malassimilation* – due to maldigestion or malabsorption of nutrients
- *Malutilisation* – nutrients are digested and absorbed normally but are utilised abnormally by the body.

It is important to have a basic understanding of the normal physiology of nutrient assimilation to appreciate the rationale for this diagnostic approach.

Normal physiology

There are three phases of assimilation of nutrients – any phase may be perturbed resulting in malassimilation.

Lumenal:

- enzyme *secretion* (primarily pancreatic) into the gut lumen
- *digestive activity* within the gut lumen

Mucosal:

- digestive activity of the mucosal cell surface
- absorption of nutrients into the mucosal cell
- any processing of nutrients within the mucosal cell

Delivery:

- transfer of nutrients from the mucosal cell into the blood

Maldigestion

Animals with maldigestion will usually present with grossly abnormal faeces and significant weight loss, despite a normal or often greatly increased appetite. The most common cause of maldigestion is exocrine pancreatic insufficiency (EPI) – other disorders occur infrequently or are just one component of a disease pathophysiology.

Examples include the following:

- Secondary enzyme deficiency resulting when luminal conditions are not optimal for enzyme function, for example inactivation of pancreatic enzymes due to gastric acid hypersecretion
- Loss of or impaired bile salts activity due to ileal or liver disease
- Brush border enzyme deficiency
    - Congenital
        - Trehalase (cats)
        - Aminopeptidase N (beagles)

  - Acquired enzyme loss
    - Relative lactose deficiency.

Occasionally, animals with EPI may develop large bowel diarrhoea. This may be due to the irritant effects of malassimilated fats on colonic mucosa and/or bacterial overgrowth.

Malabsorption

Malabsorption may occur if any of the phases of absorption of nutrients – luminal, mucosal or transport – are impaired. Diarrhoea is usually present but it may be subtle, and occasionally faeces may seem relatively normal.

An example of an abnormal *luminal* condition is dysmotility in hyperthyroidism resulting in rapid intestinal transit.

Abnormal *mucosal* function may involve the following:

- Deficiency of brush border protein transport. This may be congenital as in inherited selective cobalamin deficiency or acquired secondary to diffuse intestinal disease.
- Enterocyte defects that may occur for example in inflammatory bowel disease or villus atrophy

The *transport* phase may be abnormal due to the following:

- Lymphatic obstruction
  - Primary due to lymphangiectasia
  - Secondary due to obstruction caused by neoplasia, infection or inflammation
- Vascular compromise
  - Vasculitis, for example due to infection or immune mediated disease
  - Portal hypertension caused by a hepatopathy or right-sided heart failure.

4 Define the system and lesion

Reviewing the pathophysiology of malassimilation in the previous sections, it is obvious that malabsorption may be due to primary or secondary GI disease.

Primary GI

Primary GI causes of malabsorption are caused by infiltrative disease of the small bowel causing extensive damage to the intestinal wall.

Determination of the aetiology of primary GI causes of malabsorption almost always requires a gut biopsy.

Primary GI causes of malabsorption include the following:

- Inflammatory bowel disease
- Infiltrative neoplasia, for example lymphosarcoma and mast cell tumour
- Dietary intolerance/hypersensitivity
- Granulomatous FIP
- Lymphangiectasia
- Deep mycoses (in appropriate geographical areas)
- Occasionally, severe small intestinal bacterial overgrowth (SIBO) or antibiotic responsive diarrhoea (ARD) will cause clinically significant malabsorption.

Secondary GI disease

The most notable secondary GI disorders that will cause malabsorption are hyperthyroidism and hepatic disease. Hyperthyroidism causes increased faecal bulk secondary to increased food intake and a rapid gut transit time, which decreases the time available to absorb nutrients. Hepatic disease can result in maldigestion and malabsorption as a result of decreased bile salt excretion and malabsorption due to portal hypertension. In the vast majority of cases of liver disease, other clinical signs will predominate, but weight loss may appear excessive in relation to the appetite.

Malutilisation

Malutilisation syndromes are associated with weight loss, despite a normal or increased appetite. Diarrhoea is usually not a predominant feature, although it may occur with other clinical signs in some disorders such as hyperthyroidism and liver disease.

4 Define the lesion

Examples of disorders that cause malutilisation include the following:

- Diabetes mellitus
- Congestive heart failure (also component of malabsorption involved)
- Dirofilariasis (in endemic areas)

- Neoplasia (due to secretion of cachectin?)
- Hyperthyroidism
- Liver disease

  Animals with liver disease will usually have a reduced appetite, but it can be relatively normal and occasionally increased if the patient is not nauseous. It has been demonstrated that people with acute liver disease can become highly catabolic with marked increases in energy expenditure and therefore experience significant weight loss if increased calories are not consumed. Significant alterations in metabolism leading to early recruitment of alternate fuel sources and accelerated catabolism are reported in people, as well as a shift to muscle protein and adipose tissue utilisation. While the metabolism of animals with liver disease has not been studied as thoroughly, significant weight loss greater than that expected for the nutrient input is often clinically observed in these patients.
- Renal disease

  Animals with glomerular renal disease may lose weight due to protein loss in the urine, although this needs to be marked and is usually accompanied by systemic signs of hypoproteinaemia. Most animals with tubular renal disease lose weight because of a *reduced* appetite, but the diagnosis should be considered in a patient with weight loss despite an apparently normal appetite, as the appetite may decline so gradually and subtly that the owner does not really notice and considers that their pet is eating relatively normally. Combined with the catabolic effect of renal protein loss and skeletal muscle wasting, these patients can present with significant weight loss (but will *not* have an *increased* appetite).

Concurrent clinical signs and the history will usually assist the clinician in narrowing the focus for diagnostic procedures. Note that some disorders usually cause true polyphagia (e.g. diabetes mellitus and hyperthyroidism), whereas others do not actually increase in appetite – rather, they are associated with weight loss despite a normal appetite (e.g. heart failure, heart worm disease, neoplasia and renal disease). They may also cause a reduced appetite, in which case, the degree of weight loss can seem more marked than expected for the degree of inappetance.

In conclusion

Weight loss is a relatively common clinical sign that may be the prime focus of the case assessment, or it may be a consequence of other more specific problems. Remember that if diarrhoea is an important clinical feature, incorporate the diagnostic approaches discussed in the chapter on diarrhoea as appropriate. A history of persistent diarrhoea will usually indicate that maldigestion or malabsorption is most likely but, in cats particularly, consider hyperthyroidism. The only practically relevant cause of maldigestion (not associated with other clinical signs) is EPI, which can be diagnosed by determining plasma trypsin-like immunoreactivity (TLI) levels. Remember that hyperthyroidism and hepatic disease can cause a degree of malabsorption and hence increased faecal fat content.

Serum biochemistry and haematology may give peripheral information about the type of GI pathology causing malabsorption but cannot provide a specific tissue diagnosis. Blood tests, however, may be useful to rule out causes of malutilisation – always consider hyperthyroidism in cats and request a T4 when appropriate.

If maldigestion, malutilisation and secondary GI causes of malabsorption have been ruled out, malabsorption due to primary GI disease must be occurring – a gut biopsy (via endoscopy or laparotomy) is usually now needed to establish the diagnosis.

CHAPTER 5
Abdominal enlargement

Jill E. Maddison
The Royal Veterinary College, Department of Clinical Science and Services, London, UK

An enlarged abdomen may be an obvious clinical sign and the reason the animal is presented to the veterinarian. Or it may be a finding during the clinical examination. As with many clinical signs, the causes of abdominal enlargement range from clinically innocuous to life threatening, and a robust structured approach to its assessment is crucial.

1 Define the problem

Abdominal enlargement may be due to the intra-abdominal presence of fluid but also due to gas or solid material or to weakness of the abdominal musculature causing apparent enlargement.

Remembering the five 'F's' is a good starting point:

- Fluid
- Fat
- Flatus – for example gastric torsion
- Faeces
- Foetus

In addition, significant enlargement of intra-abdominal organs (spleen and liver) or the presence of tumour masses may also cause abdominal enlargement.

A 'pot-bellied' appearance is common in dogs with hyperadrenocorticism due to a combination of factors – abdominal muscle weakness, redistribution of fat and hepatomegaly.

The presence of an abdominal effusion *per se* rarely disrupts organ function. This is in contrast to pleural effusion which will usually

Clinical Reasoning in Small Animal Practice, First Edition.
Jill E. Maddison, Holger A. Volk and David B. Church.

cause significant and sometimes life threatening disruption of respiratory function as the normal expansion of the lungs is restricted.

Diagnostic procedures to identify the cause of the abdominal enlargement might include abdominal imaging and abdominocentesis. Once the problem is defined, that is the substance causing abdominal enlargement has been identified, then the diagnostic approach to progress to a diagnosis is usually reasonably clear. We will now concentrate on the problem of abdominal enlargement caused by fluid accumulation, as it is here that certain steps are important to further refine the problem and go on to define the system involved and lesion.

1 Refine the problem

If the cause of the abdominal enlargement is confirmed as being due to the presence of intra-abdominal fluid, then characterisation of the fluid is crucial in guiding further diagnostic steps. Patients with abdominal effusion will often have noticeable (to the owner and/or veterinarian) abdominal enlargement and a detectable 'fluid wave'. Frequently, however, such enlargement is automatically assessed to be due to 'ascites' and therapy initiated without further identification of the cause. Diagnostic tools needed to classify fluids are relatively simple. They include gross examination and measurement of specific gravity and protein content (using a refractometer) and examination of a stained smear (can be done in the house or at a laboratory depending on tools and expertise available).

Fluid characterisation

Abdominal fluid may be broadly classified as follows:

- Haemorrhagic
- Urine
- Transudate
- Modified transudate
- Exudate

- Eosinophilic
- Chyle
- Cystic fluid (if a cystic structure is sampled)

Where is the fluid?

The distribution of the fluid may be useful in narrowing down the possible causes:

- The presence of both abdominal and pleural effusion suggests generalised disease, for example heart failure, hypoproteinaemia, coagulopathy and FIP.
- Fluid confined to one cavity could be due to any of the above-mentioned as well as more localised pathology.
- If subcutaneous oedema is also present, hypoproteinaemia is most probable.

The first step in establishing a diagnosis is to classify the type of fluid present – it is not always an exact science, but more often than not it will assist in narrowing down the list of diagnostic possibilities.

Ascites

Ascites is defined as the abnormal accumulation of transudate or modified transudate in the peritoneal cavity. Portal hypertension (due to various causes) is the most common cause of ascites.

Pure transudate

- Low cellularity (<0.5–1.0×10^9 cells/L)
- Primary cell type is mononuclear cells
- Protein <25–30 g/L
- Specific gravity <1.018

Modified transudate

- Higher cellularity (up to 5.0×10^9 cells/L)
- Increased numbers of neutrophils
- Protein up to 35 g/L
- The fluid may appear serosanguinous (i.e. contains some RBCs)
- Specific gravity 1.018–1.025

A modified transudate is, as the name suggests, a transudate the characteristics of which have been modified by time within the abdominal cavity, and thus the causes are the same as a transudate.

Causes of transudates

Portal hypertension

Portal hypertension can be classified based on the location of portal blood flow restriction into the following:

- Prehepatic hypertension
- Intrahepatic presinusoidal portal hypertension
- Posthepatic obstruction

Prehepatic hypertension

Prehepatic hypertension is an uncommon cause of ascites, because if the portal vein is obstructed, lymph flow from the bowel dramatically increases and compensates for obstructed portal vein drainage. In addition, collateral communications open up between the portal system and the caudal vena cava.

Causes include the following:

- Blockage to portal vein flow by stenosis
- Portal vein thrombosis
- Extrinsic compression of the portal vein by abscesses, neoplasms or enlarged lymph nodes in the porta hepatis.

Liver size is usually normal, and the ascites has a low protein content (<25 g/L).

Intrahepatic portal hypertension

Intrahepatic portal hypertension can occur in the following conditions:

- Hepatic arteriovenous fistulas
  - uninhibited inflow of arterial blood into the portal system increases blood flow through the liver and elevates the hydrostatic portal vein pressure
- Chronic active hepatitis
- Liver cirrhosis and fibrosis
- Intrahepatic neoplasia
- Severe fatty infiltration

The liver size can be normal, increased or decreased, and the protein content of the ascites is variable.

Posthepatic obstruction

This is the most common type of portal hypertension.

Causes include the following:

- Right heart failure
- Pericardial disease
- Right atrial neoplasms
- Thrombosis or extrinsic compression of the caudal vena cava or hepatic veins, for example by neoplasms

  Because the pressure in the caudal vena cava is elevated at the same time as portal vein pressure, there is no gradient between the two systems and no collaterals form to decompress the elevated portal pressure.

The ascitic fluid in these cases has a relatively high protein content (>25 g/L), because it is derived from protein-rich hepatic lymph. The total protein concentration of the ascitic fluid usually approximates the serum albumin concentration.

Usually, the liver size is increased, and ascites and pleural effusion are often present concurrently, contrary to the isolated ascites that occurs with intrahepatic or prehepatic portal hypertension.

Hypoproteinaemia

Hypoproteinaemia alone is rarely the sole cause of ascites. Sinusoidal epithelial cells in the liver form an extremely porous membrane, which is almost completely permeable to macromolecules, including plasma proteins. In contrast, splanchnic capillaries have a pore size 50–100 times less than that of the hepatic sinuosoids. As a consequence, the trans-sinusoidal oncotic pressure gradient in the liver is virtually zero, while it is 0.8–0.9 (80–90% of maximum) in the splanchnic circulation.

Oncotic pressure gradients at such extreme ends of the spectrum minimise any effect the changes in plasma albumin concentration may have on transmicrovascular fluid exchange. Therefore, the old concept that ascites is formed secondary to decreased oncotic pressure is false, and plasma albumin concentrations have little influence on the rate of ascites formation. In patients with liver disease, portal hypertension is critical to the development of ascites, and ascites rarely develops in patients with a wedged hepatic venous portal gradient of less than 12 mm Hg.

When hypoproteinaemia is the result of chronic liver disease or glomerular disease, avid sodium retention via an undefined mechanism occurs. Avid sodium retention results in fluid retention and hence ascites. The mechanism may involve activation of the renin-angiotensin-aldosterone system, deficiency of atrial natiuretic factor or changes in intrarenal blood flow under the regulation of intrarenal prostaglandins. In addition, in the case of hepatic cirrhosis, hepatic venous outflow obstruction causes a rise in portal venous pressure and hepatic sinusoidal perfusion pressure.

Ascites as a result of hypoproteinaemia alone usually does not occur until the albumin concentration is less than 15 g/L and usually less than 10 g/L. Thus, if ascites is present in a hypoproteinaemic animal but the albumin concentration is greater than 15 g/L, hepatic or glomerular disease is more probable than protein-losing enteropathy, as avid sodium retention (and thus fluid) occurs in both glomerular and hepatic disease.

Lymphatic obstruction

Obstruction of lymphatic flow, for example by neoplasms or a diaphragmatic hernia can cause ascites.

Exudates

Characteristics

- Usually high cellularity (>5.0 × 10^9 cells/L); however, some exudates may have only moderate cellularity (e.g. FIP exudates and neoplastic exudates)
- Cell type is neutrophils and mononuclear cells
  - In *non-septic exudates,* the neutrophils are non-degenerative, and there is no evidence of organisms. The fluid may appear serosanguinous (i.e. contains some red blood cells)
  - In *septic exudates,* the nucleated cell count is extremely high, degenerate neutrophils are the predominant cells and bacteria can often be observed within neutrophils and macrophages.
- Protein >30 g/L
- Specific gravity >1.025
- Cystic fluid (e.g. hydronephrosis) may also have the characteristics of a non-septic exudate, that is high protein and moderate to high cellularity (the cells may be degenerating and look aged).

Causes of non-septic exudates

- Bile peritonitis
  - Initially non-septic but soon becomes septic if rupture is associated with biliary tract necrosis
  - In traumatic biliary rupture, bile is initially sterile but causes changes in mucosal permeability leading to secondary bacterial infection
  - The patient will be jaundiced
- FIP
  - Often contains fibrin strands, and cellularity may or may not be particularly high
- Neoplasia
- Non-septic peritonitis
  - for example secondary to pancreatitis
- Chronic inflammatory hepatopathies
- Diaphragmatic hernia
- Steatitis
- Urine peritonitis

Causes of septic exudates

- Peritonitis
  - Penetrating abdominal wound
  - Bowel perforation
  - Bile peritonitis

Eosinophilic effusions

Characteristics

Eosinophilic effusions have the characteristics of either a transudate or exudate, but in addition, greater than 10% of the cells are eosinophils.

Causes

- Aberrant larval migrans
- Mast cell tumour
- Lymphoma
- Fungal disease
- Disseminated eosinophilic granulomatosis

Blood

To confirm that blood obtained by abdomino- or thoracocentesis has not come from a 'normal' vessel or the heart, check to see if the sample clots after withdrawal. If it does not (and the animal does not have a bleeding disorder), then the blood has been free in the abdomen or thorax for sufficient time to defibrinate (usually >1 h). If the blood clots, then you have probably inadvertently tapped a vascular organ or blood vessel.

Haemorrhagic effusions initially have a similar cellular distribution to peripheral blood, although neutrophils and macrophages will increase in number with time. Erythrophagocytosis is often present, which can also assist in distinguishing true haemorrhagic effusion from traumatic collection.

Animals with intra-abdominal haemorrhage as a result of a ruptured neoplastic spleen will often be polydipsic (and polyuric with a urine SG of any value).

Causes

Haemoabdomen can be due to intra-abdominal disease (e.g. bleeding neoplasm such as splenic haemangiosarcoma, fracture of liver or spleen, avulsion of renal arteries or iatrogenic postoperatively) or systemic disorders such as a coagulopathy (discussed in Chapter 11).

Urine

The presence of urine throughout the abdomen can be due to the bladder being large and flaccid or a ruptured bladder. If uncertain about whether fluid obtained from an abdominal tap is urine or an effusion (very dilute urine can grossly look the same as a transudate), measure the urea or creatinine concentration. If it is urine, it should be substantially higher than the plasma concentration. If it is an effusion, the concentration will be about the same as plasma. However, this is usually useful only during the first 24 h after bladder rupture, as after this, equilibrium develops between the peritoneal fluid and serum, thus reducing the diagnostic value of this test.

Chyle

Chyle is triglyceride-rich fluid that leaks into the thoracic or peritoneal cavity from the thoracic duct or intestinal lymphatics.

Characteristics

- Remains opaque when centrifuged
- Protein = 20–60 g/L
- Specific gravity >1.018
- Cellularity – $0.4–10.0 \times 10^9$ cells/L
- Cell type
  - early in the disease, predominantly small lymphocytes with few neutrophils
  - later, non-degenerate neutrophils become more predominant, there are fewer lymphocytes, macrophages increase in number and plasma cells may be present.
- The fluid clears when ether is added (which dissolves the chylomicrons)
- The triglyceride concentration is greater than that in serum, and the cholesterol concentration is less than that in serum
- Cholesterol: triglyceride ratio < 1
- Sudanophilic fat globules are present
- Pseudochylous effusion looks similar to chyle but does not have the aforementioned characteristics
- The relevance of differentiating pseudochylous from chylous effusion is questionable – as they are both caused by a similar range of pathologies, differentiation does not assist in narrowing down the list of possible causes.

Causes

- Lymphangiectasia
- Obstruction or rupture of lymphatics due to neoplasia
- Right-sided heart failure

In conclusion

The key to assessing the patient with abdominal enlargement is to first confirm what is causing the enlargement. If fluid is detected, then it is relatively easy to classify the type of fluid present, which then permits generation of a rational differential list. But remember, there are overlaps in differentials, and as often in clinical medicine, the picture isn't always clear cut. So all information gathered from the history, clinical examination, fluid analysis, laboratory tests and diagnostic imaging is valuable in helping reach a diagnosis.

CHAPTER 6
Weakness

Holger A. Volk[1], David B. Church[2] & Jill E. Maddison[1]
[1] *The Royal Veterinary College, Department of Clinical Science and Services, London, UK*
[2] *The Royal Veterinary College, London, UK*

Weakness is a common presenting complaint in general practice. It is always a sign of central nervous system (CNS) or neuromuscular system dysfunction, and hence the answer to the question 'what system or systems *must* be involved' in a patient presenting with weakness is always going to be the CNS or neuromuscular system. This involvement can be either primary, that is due to abnormalities of some part of the CNS or the neuromuscular system itself, or secondary, where its dysfunction is brought about by the consequences of abnormalities of another body system or systems. Primary causes are frequently going to result in structural changes to the CNS or neuromuscular system and may result in focal or localised exacerbated dysfunction, while secondary problems do not result in structural changes and their effects are usually more generalised. This chapter provides you with a toolkit to refine the potential diagnoses to those that are more common. Even if the underlying aetiology is not 100% defined, this can allow you to give the owner some answers about probable causes and prognosis.

Initial assessment of the weak patient

1 Define the problem

When an animal presents with a history of episodic weakness, fatigability or collapse, appropriately defining the problem is essential, although sometimes difficult. An owner may state that their dog

Clinical Reasoning in Small Animal Practice, First Edition.
Jill E. Maddison, Holger A. Volk and David B. Church.

is having collapsing episodes, but it is imperative that the clinician defines the problem by gathering the following key information:

- What happens before or after the episode?
- What was observed during the episode?
- Does the animal lose consciousness during the episode? (seen in syncope or seizures).

This will enable the clinician to ascertain whether:

- The animal loses *consciousness* (indicating syncope or seizures).
- There is *no* evidence of *convulsive* activity (more likely syncope than seizures).
- The animal is normal in between the episodes (*episodically weak*), whether weakness is precipitated by exercise (*fatigability*) or the animal is consistently weak (*persistently weak*).
- The animal shows a *spastic* or *flaccid* 'weakness' associated with or without incoordination (*ataxia*).

Other common presenting complaints that may be seen in the flaccidly weak patient include the following:

- Regurgitation
- Paresis
- Difficulty rising
- Exercise intolerance
- Episodic weakness
- Fatigability
- Altered voice
- Change in musculature
- Stiff stilted gait
- An inability to lift the head up normally or, especially in cats, a state of persistent cervical ventroflexion.

Musculoskeletal disorders

Skeletal disorders involving joint or bone pathology may be confused with weakness due to neurological disease (also see Chapter 13). Examples would include dogs with bilateral cruciate rupture presented for pelvic limb 'paralysis' and animals with lumbosacral disease presented for pelvic limb weakness. As a result, it is vitally important that before embarking on a diagnostic work up for a neurological problem (structural or functional), skeletal disorders are considered and ruled out where appropriate. Also keep in mind that a patient may have concurrent skeletal and CNS or neuromuscular system disorders such as the German Shepherd dog with a pelvic limb gait abnormality contributed to by hip-dysplasia-induced degenerative joint disease *and* degenerative myelopathy (also see Chapter 13).

2 Define the system

Animals with dysfunction of the CNS or neuromuscular system can present collapsed or weak. The nervous system is divided into the CNS (brain and spinal cord) and the neuromuscular system (peripheral nerves, neuromuscular junction and musculature). The CNS regulates the neuromuscular system. The cause either can be a primary, structural disorder of the CNS or neuromuscular system or can result from the dysfunction of a number of other systems that result in impaired CNS or neuromuscular function.

This dysfunction can result in impaired CNS or neuromuscular performance in a number of different ways including the following:

- Reduced delivery of nutrients to the brain, nerves or muscles
  - for example glucose and oxygen
- Impaired vascular function
  - for example polycythaemia and hyperglobulinaemia
- Change in the internal milieu of muscles and nerves that alter their function
  - for example calcium and potassium imbalances
- Production of endogenous toxins
  - for example uraemia.

Hence, it is apparent that weakness may be caused by:

- Primary, structural CNS or neuromuscular disease involving the following:
  - Brain
  - Spinal cord
  - Peripheral nerves
  - Neuromuscular junction
  - Muscles
- Secondary, functional CNS and/or neuromuscular disease caused by:
  - Cardiovascular/haematopoietic disorders
    - heart, vessels and blood

- Metabolic disorders
  - electrolytes
  - glucose
  - endogenous toxins
- Respiratory disorders
- Skeletal disorders.

Animals presenting with a more flaccid weakness must have a problem with their neuromuscular system, and this is discussed in this chapter. See Chapter 7 for the detailed clinical reasoning approach for animals presenting with the primary sign of 'collapse' and Chapter 13 for the detailed clinical reasoning approach for animals presenting with the primary complaint of a combination of gait abnormalities, a more spastic 'weakness' (upper motor neuron paresis) and/or incoordination of movement (ataxia).

3 Define the location

In CNS or neuromuscular disorders causing weakness, the clinical and neurological examination is the key in determining the system involved and, when appropriate, what part of the system. The neurological examination can help you define the location of the lesion within the CNS (see Chapters 7 and 13) or neuromuscular system ('is it central or peripheral? And if central or peripheral, where is the location?'), and this in turn can assist in confirming the system involved and whether there is likely to be a structural or functional disorder.

Common neurological examination findings in neuromuscular disorders

- Tetraparesis +/– proprioceptive ataxia.
  - Paresis is a sign of motor dysfunction and ataxia of sensory nerve/proprioceptive dysfunction. In general, if you find paresis without ataxia, think 'muscular'.
- Muscle atrophy/pain
- Reduced spinal reflexes and muscle tone
- Sensory deficits or self mutilation.

In general, evidence for sensory dysfunction strongly suggests a primary neuromuscular problem, as it is unusual for a functional problem to result in predominantly sensory dysfunction.

It is also always important to check for autonomic dysfunction, as this can be associated with a range of neuropathies. Autonomic dysfunction can be manifested by changes such as the following:

- Mydriasis or anisocoria
- Decreased tear production
- Hyposalivation
- Bradycardia
- Constipation
- Urinary retention.

If you see most (only) of the aforementioned autonomic deficits, you might have a primary problem of the autonomic nervous system (e.g. feline or canine dysautonomia).

Neuroanatomical localisation within the CNS or neuromuscular system

The neurological examination can be divided into two parts (see also Chapter 7):

1. Hands-off examination – observation
   - Mentation and behaviour
   - Posture
   - Gait
   - Identification of abnormal involuntary movements (Chapter 7)
2. Hands-on examination
   - Postural reaction testing
   - Cranial nerves assessment
   - Spinal reflexes, muscle tone and size
   - Sensory evaluation.

Hands-off examination – Observation

Mentation and behaviour

The most important part is the hands-off examination. The first thing you always need to assess and ask the owner about is if the animal has developed or shows an abnormal behaviour and has a change in mentation (e.g. obtundation). If you see changes in behaviour or an altered level of mentation, then consider brain involvement (Chapter 7). Conditions affecting purely the neuromuscular system should not cause an altered mentation or behaviour changes.

Posture and gait

Observe the animal from a distance (from the front or back [walking towards or away from you] and passing by from the side). *Ataxia* is a lack of coordination of movement and may occur in conditions affecting sensory (proprioceptive) pathways. *Paresis* is defined as a *decrease* of voluntary movement; *plegia,* on the other hand, is characterised by an *absence* of voluntary movement. Spastic (upper motor neuron) paresis or plegia occurs with disease affecting the neuronal pathways cranial to the intumescence for the limbs being affected and can be seen with CNS involvement (see Chapter 13 for details). Flaccid paresis (lower motor neuron) occurs with disorders causing loss of function of the motor unit (some part of the collective that includes the intumescence [origin of the nerves for the limb], neuromuscular junction and the related muscle or muscles). Flaccid paresis is therefore an indication of the neuromuscular system being affected. Most of the conditions will affect all four limbs, with the pelvic limbs usually being more severely affected, as they have the longer neuromuscular pathways. To identify if the muscles, the neuromuscular junctions or the peripheral nerves are affected, think 'physiologically'. Most peripheral nerves are mixed nerves having sensory and motor tracts. Thus, if they are affected, you can see ataxia and paresis (have a look at Table 6.1, and see which other deficits occur because of sensory loss). Neuromuscular junction deficits and muscle disease only cause paresis, which can resemble an orthopaedic lameness. Ataxia is best appreciated when the animal is walked slowly. Paresis in neuromuscular conditions can get worse with exercise, so also assess the animal trotting.

Hands-on examination

Postural reactions

Postural reaction tests can be helpful to confirm which limbs you think are affected. They are not so useful to determine which part of the nervous system is affected, as they are more similar to a 'screening test', testing the afferent proprioceptive (sensory) and efferent motor pathways (receptor → peripheral nerve → spinal cord → brain → spinal cord → motor unit; see also Chapter 13).

Table 6.1 Neuroanatomical localisation within the neuromuscular system. Neurological deficits to be considered with neuromuscular disease.

Neurological examination	Peripheral neuropathy	Polyradiculoneuropathy (motor)	Junctionopathy	Myopathy
Mentation	Appropriate level and quality	Appropriate level and quality	Appropriate level and quality	Appropriate level and quality
Posture/gait	Plantigrade stance Flaccid paresis or plegia of affected limb(s) (motor impairment) Ataxia (sensory impairment)	Flaccid paresis or plegia of affected limb(s)	Usually unremarkable (without exercise) Exercise-induced stiff stilted gait then/or Flaccid paresis or plegia of affected limbs (during exercise or for sever phenotype)	Stiff stilted gait (often aggravates with exercise) Paresis
Postural reactions	Postural reaction deficits on affected limb(s) (sensory and/or motor)	Postural reaction deficits on affected limbs (motor part impaired)	Unaltered to altered depending on severity of disease or exercise level	Usually unaltered Can be altered with severe phenotype or exercise
Spinal reflexes	Decreased to absent on affected limb(s)	Absent to reduced on affected limbs	Unremarkable unless severe phenotype or exercised	Unremarkable

(*continued overleaf*)

Table 6.1 *(continued)*

Neurological examination	Peripheral neuropathy	Polyradiculoneuropathy (motor)	Junctionopathy	Myopathy
Muscle tone and mass	Reduced to absent muscle tone with moderate to severe muscle atrophy (motor)	Reduced to absent muscle tone with moderate to severe muscle atrophy when chronic (motor)	Usually unremarkable	Atrophy or hypertrophy Reduced tone or contractures (hypertonicity – myotonia)
Sensation	With sensory nerve involvement decreased to absent sensation and nociception	Unremarkable	Unremarkable	Unremarkable
Cranial nerves	Can be involved	Unremarkable	Facial weakness possible	Masticatory muscle atrophy possible
Pain	Paraesthesia, self-mutilation	Spinal pain possible	Unremarkable	Possible muscle pain (e.g. inflammatory/infectious and neoplastic diseases)
Others	Autonomic signs possible			

Cranial nerve examination

CNS or neuromuscular diseases can affect the cranial nerves. The most important cranial nerve test to perform is the menace response, which tests most of the brain compartments and can be seen as a 'screening test' (retina → optic nerve → optic chiasma (about 65–75% of the fibres cross) → optic tract → lateral geniculate nucleus → optic radiation → occipital lobe of cerebrum → projections fibres → motor cortex → cerebellum → facial nucleus → facial nerve → orbicularis oculi muscle).

If the menace response is reduced or absent, then you firstly need to assess vision by seeing if the animal bumps into things when walking around. You can also test parts of the vision pathway by evaluating the pupillary light reflex (PLR). Pupil size and the presence of anisocoria should be noted before performing the PLR. Subtle anisocorias are best assessed by illuminating both eyes of the animal from a distance and looking for the tapetal reflection. It is also important, especially in elderly patients, to recognise iris atrophy, as this could falsely be recognised as anisocoria. The pathway for the PLR starts off as the menace response pathway but includes only the brainstem (retina → optic nerve → optic chiasma (about 65–75% of the fibres cross) → optic tract → pretectal nucleus → caudal comissure (most of the fibres cross again) → parasympathetic nucleus of the occulomotor nerve (cranial nerve III) → occulomotor nerve → iris sphincter).

If a patient with impaired menace response appears to have normal vision and PLR, then their ability to blink should be assessed using the palpebral reflex. The palpebral test is the most useful test for assessing the motor function of the facial nerve (CN VII) and when repeated rapidly can become diminished in patients with neuromuscular junction disorders. The sensory part of the palpebral reflex is mediated by the trigeminal nerve (CN V). In general, the trigeminal nerve has motor and sensory function. The motor part (mandibular branch) innervates all muscles of mastication; the sensory innervates the whole face (via the mandibular, maxillary and ophthalmic branches). When assessing facial sensation, reflexive (palpebral reflex) and conscious (aversive) responses can be noted.

Apart from its motor function, the facial nerve also has sensory and autonomic functions. The facial nerve innervates the muscles of facial expression. The nostril is smaller on the side of the dysfunction, the lip may drop and or a pocket of saliva can be found on the affected side. Schirmer tear test can be used to assess the tear production (an autonomic function of the facial nerve).

Asymmetry of the muscles of the head can suggest motor dysfunction of a number of cranial nerves and is best assessed from a distance.

Other cranial nerves that can be affected by CNS or neuromuscular disorders are CN IX-XII.

- Cranial nerve IX: the glossopharyngeal nerve supplies the pharynx with sensory and motor fibres. It can be assessed by the gag reflex.
- Cranial nerve X: the vagal nerve innervates the larynx and carries parasympathetic fibres for thoracic and abdominal organs.
- Cranial nerve XI: accessory nerve innervates part of the neck musculature.
- Cranial nerve XII: the hypoglossus nerve function can be assessed by observation. The tongue should be watched for any evidence of paresis, deviation, atrophy or asymmetry.

Spinal reflexes

In assessing spinal reflexes, a standard approach facilitates the clinician's capacity to detect abnormalities. Generally, changes in muscle tone should be assessed first and then the spinal reflexes themselves. Muscle tone can be reduced in neuromuscular disorders. Reflexes may also be attenuated due to muscle fibrosis or joint contractures or appear exaggerated if there is a lack of antagonistic muscle tone (pseudohyperreflexia seen with sciatic nerve lesion). Reflexes should be, therefore, interpreted only in light of the rest of the examination (gait, posture and muscle tone). In neuromuscular conditions, the reflexes are usually decreased in the affected limbs (it can be useful to assess the animal before and after exercise):

- Decreased or absent reflexes are caused by a lesion in the reflex arc (receptor → peripheral nerve → spinal cord → peripheral nerve → neuromuscular junction → muscle).
    - Decrease in tendon reflexes such as patellar reflex (reduced level of stifle extension) or biceps, triceps or gastrocnemius reflex (decrease in muscle contraction of the muscle).

- Decreased withdrawal (flexor) reflexes are shown as reduction in the degree of flexion of individual joints.
  - Pelvic limbs assessment: reduced → hock flexion (sciatic dysfunction)
  - Thoracic limbs assessment: reduced elbow flexion.

Palpation

Palpation can help you to detect muscle atrophy or hypertrophy, swelling, pain, masses, muscle contractures and muscle tone. Palpation should be done when the animal is standing and in lateral recumbency.

Sensory evaluation

Assessment of sensation can be helpful if you think the neuromuscular deficits are caused by peripheral nerve dysfunction. It is, however, rare that the animals will have severe nociceptive deficits with conditions affecting the neuromuscular system.

Neuromuscular system deficits that can be seen with defects in the different parts of the neuromuscular system can be seen in Table 6.1.

As well as considering the results of your clinical and neurological examination, think pathophysiologically to determine which body system is involved, that is consider the function of each body system and how disturbances of its function might manifest clinically. For example, it is obvious that if an animal is persistently weak and has episodes of loss of consciousness, primary muscle disease is unlikely (see 'collapse' in Chapter 7).

If the neurological deficits are asymmetrical, a primary structural CNS or neuromuscular abnormality becomes far more likely (Tables 6.2 and 6.3). If the condition is also painful, then there should be an increased index of suspicion for inflammatory, infectious, traumatic or neoplastic conditions. Secondary functional lesions affect the neuromuscular system diffusely so that the neurological deficits are usually symmetrical in presentation. For these conditions, pain cannot be elicited from structures in the neuromuscular system.

Table 6.2 Potential diagnoses for episodic or exercise induced weakness.

Category	Differentials	Symmetry of neuromuscular deficits	Pain
Secondary (functional) neuromuscular			
Cardiovascular/haematopoietic	Structural cardiovascular disease	S	–
	Arrhythmias	S	–
	Anaemia	S	–
	Hyperviscosity syndromes	S	–
	Acute haemorrhage	S	–
Respiratory	Heartworm disease	S	–
	Upper respiratory dysfunction (laryngeal paralysis, brachycephalic airway syndrome and tracheal collapse)	S	–
	Pulmonary disease	S	–
Metabolic	Hypoglycaemia (e.g. pancreatic islet tumour and exercise induced)	S	–
	Hyperkalaemia, for example hypoadrenocorticism	S	–/+
Primary (structural) CNS or neuromuscular			
Neuropathy	Exercise-induced collapse (CNS)	S	–
Junctionopathy	Myasthenia gravis	S	–
Myopathy	Metabolic myopathies (e.g. mitochondrial or lipidstorage myopathy); malignant hyperthermia	S	–

S = symmetrical neuromuscular deficits.

4 Define the lesion

You have now localised the lesion to the CNS or neuromuscular system and potentially to a specific part within this system. It is now time to identify the lesion. Questions that might help you to refine your

Table 6.3 Potential diagnoses for persistent weakness.

Category	Differentials	Symmetry of neuromuscular deficits	Pain
Secondary (functional) neuromuscular			
Cardiovascular/ haematopoietic	Cardiovascular disease	S	–
	Arrhythmias	S	–
	Anaemia	S	–
	Hyperviscosity syndromes	S	–
Metabolic	Hypokalaemia (e.g. primary aldosteronism)	S	–
	Hyperkalaemia (e.g. hypoadrenocorticism)	S	–/+
	Hypocalcaemia (e.g. primary hypoparathyroidism)	S	–/+
	Hypercalcaemia (e.g. primary hyperparathyroidism, paraneoplastic syndrome and Vitamin D toxicity)	S	–
	Hypo-/hypermagnesaemia	S	–
	Hypoglycaemia (e.g. insulinoma and hunting dog)	S	–
	Hyperadrenocorticism	S	–/+
	Hypothyroidism	S/AS	–
	Endogenous toxaemia (e.g. sepsis and hepatic encephalopathy)	S	–
Neoplasia	Paraneoplastic (e.g. insulinoma causing neuropathy)	S	–
Nutritional	Vitamine E/Selenium deficiency	S	–
Toxic	Lead (neuropathy)	S	–
	Organophosphate toxicity, spider bite, tick paralysis, botulism and snake envenomation		–
Primary (structural) CNS or neuromuscular			
Neuropathy	*Non-inflammatory*	AS	+/–
	Acquired	S	+/–
	Neoplasia (e.g. lymphoma)	AS	+/–
	Inherited	S	+/–
	Breed-specific myopathy (e.g. Alaskan Malamute and Leonberger)	AS	–

(*continued overleaf*)

Table 6.3 (*continued*)

Category	Differentials	Symmetry of neuromuscular deficits	Pain
	Inflammatory		–
	Infectious	AS	–
	Protozoal	AS	–
	Immune mediated	AS	–
	Polyradiculoneuritis	S/AS	–
	Chronic neuritis	AS	–
Junctionopathy	Myasthenia gravis	S	–
Myopathy	*Non-inflammatory*		–
	Acquired		–
	Exertional rhabdomyolysis	S	+
	Neoplasia (e.g. lymphoma)	AS	+/–
	Paraneoplastic	S	–
	Inherited		
	Muscular dystrophy	AS	+
	Myotonia	S	–
	Metabolic myopathies	S	–
	Breed-specific myopathy (e.g. Great Dane and Labrador)	S	–
	Inflammatory		
	Infectious		
	Protozoal	AS	+/–
	Rickettsial	AS	+/–
	Immune-mediated		
	Polymyositis	AS	+/–
	Dermatomyositis	AS	+/–

S = symmetrical neuromuscular deficits, AS = asymmetrical neuromuscular deficits.

list of possible diagnoses and help you consider the most appropriate diagnostic pathway are the following:

- Which diseases have a direct (primary) or indirect (secondary) effect on the CNS or neuromuscular system?
- Which diseases cause lateralising (asymmetrical) signs or symmetrical signs?
- Which disease processes could be associated with pain?
- What is the clinical course of the disease (acute vs. chronic onset; improving, static, episodic and/or deteriorating)?

- Apart from weakness, what other clinical signs do you recognise, which could indicate secondary involvement of the CNS or neuromuscular system?
  - Cardiac disease? (e.g. arrhythmias, pulse deficits, changes in pulse quality and peripheral blood perfusion problems)
  - Upper respiratory disease? (e.g. stridor, respiratory distress and clinical signs of reduced oxygenation)
  - Lower respiratory disease? (e.g. abnormal thoracic auscultation [pulmonary? pleural effusion?])
  - Endocrinopathy? (e.g. skin and haircoat changes, changes in body conformation and abdominal wall weakness)
  - Haematological disorders? (e.g. changes in mucous membrane colour and heart sounds)
  - Gastrointestinal changes (e.g. vomiting vs. regurgitation [Chapter 2])
  - Hyperthermia vs. pyrexia?

In addition, the characteristics of the weakness will assist in refining the list of possible diagnoses. As discussed earlier when defining the problem, weakness can present episodically or persistently. Exercise can trigger an episode and aggravate some of the causes of episodic weakness progressing to persistent weakness.

Weakness in cats

Cats, in contrast to dogs, do not tend to present with episodic weakness – they will usually 'self-regulate' their activity and more commonly present with persistent weakness. This is usually manifested by ventral flexion of the neck and lying with their head on their paws (i.e. looking really relaxed) even in the middle of a consulting room or other strange and stressful environments. Ventral flexion of the head is seen in cats with neuromuscular disease, as they lack a nuchal ligament. Cats also might have elevated (prominent) scapulae when they rest and walk.

Episodic weakness

Episodic weakness without loss of consciousness will usually occur with:

- Secondary functional neuromuscular disorders
  - Cardiovascular dysfunction

  - Metabolic derangements
    - energy deprivation
    - electrolyte abnormalities
- Primary structural neuromuscular disorders
  - Neuromuscular junctionopathies
    - Myasthenia gravis
  - Myopathies.

See Table 7.1 for specific examples of disorders causing episodic weakness.

Persistent weakness

Persistent weakness usually occurs with:

- Secondary functional neuromuscular disorders
  - derangements in calcium or potassium homeostasis
  - endogenous toxaemia
- Primary structural neuromuscular disorders
  - primary peripheral nerve dysfunction
  - neuromuscular junction abnormalities
  - primary muscle dysfunction.

Persistent weakness aggravated by exercise usually occurs with:

- Secondary functional neuromuscular disorders
  - Cardiovascular system disorders
  - Metabolic disorders
- Primary structural neuromuscular disorders
  - Peripheral neuropathy
  - Junctionopathy
  - Myopathy.

See Table 6.3 for specific examples of disorders causing persistent weakness.

The direction of your diagnostic procedures will depend on other clinical signs and abnormalities that are present in addition to the presenting complaint of weakness.

Diagnostic approach

Your diagnostic approach will be determined by your problem-solving path. Most of the diagnostics for diseases that affect the neuromuscular system secondarily can be performed in general practice. These include detailed history, complete physical and neurological examination, blood and urine tests, blood pressure measurements, examination of the retina (looking for convoluted and/or dilated blood vessels or bleeding, indicating signs of hypertension) and imaging modalities accessible in first opinion practice such as radiography and ultrasonography.

Diagnostic tests can be grouped into

1 Clinical pathology,
2 Assessment of structure using diagnostic imaging and/or pathology techniques and
3 Functional assessment (mainly electrodiagnostics).

Clinical pathology

Haematology, serum biochemistry and urinalysis

Routine haematology, serum biochemistry and urinalysis can be especially useful in situations where the deficits in the neuromuscular systems are generalised or symmetrical and the suspicion is for compromised function secondary to systemic problems due to other body system dysfunction. Generally, there will be indications of these other system or systems' involvement, and a thorough history and physical examination can be pivotal in uncovering the reasons for the secondary neurological dysfunction (e.g. hyperkalaemia and hypocalcaemia can cause gastrointestinal dysfunction; hypoglycaemia can also cause seizures; see Chapter 7). Timing of blood sampling can also be important, for example collect fasting blood glucose samples if hypoglycaemia is suspected (multiple samples might be needed, as autonomous insulin production can vary substantially from hour to hour and glucose can be modified by homeostatic mechanisms, e.g. stress response, cortisol). On occasions, even haematology can be helpful in providing clues regarding possible infectious and non-infectious inflammatory disorders.

Interpreting serum creatine kinase activity levels

Creatine kinase (CK) activity in serum is often measured in dogs and cats when a myopathy is suspected, as the enzyme is a relatively specific indicator of muscle damage. CK activity is not only raised with skeletal myopathies, but also raised with cardiac myopathies. Seizures have also been reported to increase CK activity secondary to muscle damage. Even relatively minor muscle damage associated, for example with a recumbent animal or with an intramuscular injection, will result in increased serum CK activity. It is therefore important not to over-interpret mild to moderate (<1000 U/L) increases in enzyme activity. Even levels greater than 1000 U/L may be associated with secondary muscle damage and are not necessarily indicative of primary muscle disease. It is also important to note that it takes a couple of hours until CK activity in the serum is increased. Thus, it is not true that CK activity will increase because the animal was difficult to handle during the bleeding procedure. For a serum CK activity to be considered truly strongly suggestive of a significant myopathy (e.g. myositis and muscular dystrophy), the concentration needs to be in the thousands to tens of thousands. It is also important to remember that not all animals with a significant myopathy will have a marked serum CK elevation, and thus, it is always worth evaluating not only CK, but also serum ALT and AST activity, as both of these enzymes may or may not be elevated in cases of severe primary myopathy.

Serology

Immune-mediated impairment of the neuromuscular junction, more commonly known as myasthenia gravis, is common compared to the other neuromuscular diseases and should be considered in every dog presented for episodic, exercise-induced generalised weakness, regurgitation, megaoesophagus or pharyngeal dysfunction. The assay for the detection of the autoantibodies directed against the post-synaptic acetylcholine receptor (AChR) has relatively high sensitivity and specificity. In cases where you suspect a myositis or neuritis, serology for the most common infectious diseases can be performed – *Neospora caninum, Toxoplasma gondii.* For a diagnosis of toxoplasmosis to be confirmed, it is essential to determine both the relevant IgG and IgM levels of toxoplasma antibodies to help differentiate between former exposure and acute infection.

Endocrine function testing

Many endocrinologic disorders, endogenous and iatrogenic, result in neuromuscular weakness (e.g. hypothyroidism, hyperadrenocorticism, hypoadrenocorticism and iatrogenic steroid myopathy).

Cerebrospinal fluid analysis

When evaluating an animal in which you suspect primary neurological disease, analysis of cerebrospinal fluid (CSF) can be considered, especially in the investigation of diseases involving the meninges or nerve roots. CSF analysis is a sensitive, but usually not specific, test; however, the results always need to be interpreted in the light of the animal's clinical presentation. The CSF analysis can help reduce the list of differential diagnoses, especially if inflammatory and infectious causes are suspected. CSF analysis must be performed very quickly after collection (usually in 30 min), as cells degrade rapidly in CSF. There are a number of techniques that stabilise the samples for longer. As these differ between laboratories, it is always wise to establish the relevant laboratory's preferred protocol before sampling.

Genetic testing

A number of primary CNS and neuromuscular disorders are brought about by gene abnormalities, and there are increasing battery of tests that allow the abnormalities to be identified. Most of them are for breed-specific diseases. Examples currently include the following:

- Polyneuropathy in Alaskan Malamute,
- Greyhound neuropathy,
- Hereditary myopathy in Labrador Retriever and Great Dane,
- Specific glycogen storage diseases in dogs and cats,
- Congenital hypothyroidism in Spanish Water dogs,
- Exercise-induced collapse,
- Fucosidosis in English Springer Spaniels,
- Familial episodic hypokalaemic polymyopathy in Burmese cats.

Assessing structural lesions

Diagnostic imaging

Radiography is a widely available and relatively inexpensive tool allowing the rapid 'screening' for obvious bony and some soft tissue abnormalities. It can help to characterise structural changes in thoracic anatomy, for example evidence of cardiomegaly or other structural heart changes, lung pattern changes, evidence of metastatic disease, mediastinal masses (e.g. thymoma) or meagoesophagus.

Computed tomography (CT) provides far better spatial resolution than radiography but is not readily available in most practices. Magnetic resonance imaging (MRI) has been shown to be an accurate technique to image muscular pathology (e.g. myositis) and peripheral nerves (e.g. nerve sheath tumours). Although ultrasonography can be useful in visualising a limited number of peripheral nerves such as the sciatic nerve, the femoral nerve and the brachial plexus, generally, its lack of precision makes it value, at best, limited.

Biopsy

A full tissue biopsy of peripheral nerve or muscle can be helpful to identify pathology when appropriately taken and processed as advised by a specialised laboratory. Histopathology and immunohistochemistry of tissues can help to differentiate many primary structural lesions, for example inflammatory, infectious vs. neoplastic conditions. Evidence of denervation, endocrinopathies, specific metabolic abnormalities such as hypokalaemia, mitochondrial myopathy, neoplasia, inflammatory/infectious conditions (myositis and neuritis), storage diseases or muscular dystrophy may be identified. Muscle biopsies are relatively easy to perform in general practice; however, peripheral nerve biopsies are more challenging. In some cases, electrodiagnostic testing can be useful before sampling to help identify the nerve and/or the muscle to be biopsied.

Functional assessment

Electrophysiology

The nervous system communicates via the generation and propagation of electrical impulses. These electrical potentials may be measured directly (spontaneous activity), or electrical stimuli can be applied to induce electrical potentials, which can be used for assessment of the integrity of tested pathways (evoked potentials). Abnormal spontaneous muscular activity may be caused either by primary disease of the muscle (e.g. myositis and muscular dystrophy) or by denervation of the muscle. Electromyography can help to assess which muscles are affected. Evoked potentials generated through stimulating a nerve (nerve conduction studies) can help to localise the lesion to a specific part of the nerve or the neuromuscular junction and help indicate axon and/or myelin loss.

Pharmacological testing of function

The short-acting anticholinesterase drug edrophonium chloride (Tensilon®) may be used to provide a presumptive diagnosis of acquired myasthenia gravis in dogs and cats. This test can elicit a cholinergic crisis and may cause salivation, retching, vomiting and diarrhoea and therefore should only be performed in a controlled setting with atropine prepared and available for administration if required. A false-positive result can occur, as other neuromuscular weaknesses can improve when edrophonium is given. The gold standard, therefore, remains the assay for autoantibodies against AChRs. The test can be very useful to assess the prognosis for the clinical response to the longer acting pyridostigmine.

Exercise test

Exercise and excitement can trigger and aggravate neuromuscular weakness. Resting and post-exercise plasma lactate (and pyruvate concentrations), CK activity levels, cardiorespiratory function (mucous membranes, pulse quality and rhythm and blood oxygenation) and temperature can be measured and help highlight subtle changes. Lactate and pyruvate level changes can indicate mitochondrial disease.

In conclusion

The patient presenting weak or collapsed can pose a significant diagnostic dilemma. Understanding the pathophysiology underlying weakness can assist the clinician follow a structured diagnostic pathway and importantly reduces the need to remember long lists of differential diagnoses. Focus on the key questions – which part of the CNS or neuromuscular system is involved and is the involvement due to primary structural or neuromuscular pathology or dysfunction secondary to some other problem resulting in neuromuscular dysfunction? If you follow these steps, you will be able to reach a refined list of possible explanations or even diagnoses rationally and expediently.

CHAPTER 7

Fit, collapse or strange episodes

Holger A. Volk
The Royal Veterinary College, Department of Clinical Science and Services, London, UK

Introduction

A patient presented with a history of paroxysmal episodes or 'fits' can provide any experienced clinician with an interesting challenge. Firstly, the patient is usually normal at presentation. Secondly, the identification of the type of episode is dependent on a good description from the person who witnessed the episode. Thirdly, most of these paroxysmal episodes appear unpredictable and uncontrollable for the owner, and therefore, their observation might be heavily biased by an emotionally loaded perception of reality. A detailed history is, however, vital before embarking on a diagnostic investigation. Many owners can video the events, which can help the clinician characterise them.

Syncope, narcolepsy/cataplexy, pain, compulsive behaviour disorders, vestibular attacks, certain movement disorders, neuromuscular weakness and seizures are paroxysmal events, which share commonalities in their clinical presentation. The inter-episodic clinical examination can be *normal* for these presentations. Some of the animals might present with *inter-episodic deficits*, and this will guide your clinical decision-making and help you determine the system involved (and localise the lesion within). The animals might even *present with the* 'strange' *episode* at your clinic, for example prolonged seizure activity (status epilepticus [>5 minutes] and cluster seizures [≥2 seizure/day]) or vestibular dysfunction.

Clinical Reasoning in Small Animal Practice, First Edition.
Jill E. Maddison, Holger A. Volk and David B. Church.

1 Define the problem

Paroxysmal episodic disorders can have many presentations affecting posture, muscle tone, uncontrolled movements and alteration in behaviour. Apart from characterising the episode itself, it is important to establish any triggers or clinical signs the animal might show before or shortly after an episode (Table 7.1). Common episodic events that need to be differentiated are syncope, narcolepsy/cataplexy, behaviour changes, vestibular attacks, movement disorders, neuromuscular weakness and seizures.

Syncope

Episodes of syncope are usually characterized by a sudden, short, transient loss of consciousness and postural tone. The animals are flaccid during the episode but can experience a brief myoclonic jerk just before collapsing. We have seen this especially in cats with 3rd degree atrioventricular block. This can be confused with brief focal seizures. However, most animals with syncopal episodes do not show any pre- or post-episodic signs. Syncopal episodes are commonly associated with exercise or movement rather than occurring at rest. Recovery is usually nearly instant. There can be multiple episodes per day, which can occur shortly after each other and show no improvement on anti-epileptic drugs. In fact, anti-epileptic drugs can impair cardiorespiratory function, and therefore, these episodes can get worse with anti-epileptic drug treatment.

Narcolepsy

Narcolepsy is a rather rare disorder of the sleep–wake cycle. Cataplectic attacks are common in narcolepsy, which can resemble syncopal collapse and seizures. Cataplectic attacks are usually triggered by food, excitement and stress or pharmacologically (e.g. physostigmine). Following the 'trigger', the affected animal will become flaccid and collapse. Narcoleptic animals experience chronic fatigue, although they do not necessarily sleep more. They can be restless at night and sleepy during the day because of a disturbed and irregular sleep pattern. A history of others affected in the litter or in the breeding line is not uncommon.

Paroxysmal behaviour changes

Pain can be experienced episodically and trigger a behavioural response, which can resemble focal seizures, for example nerve root impingement or irritation caused by lateral disc protrusion/extrusion resulting in 'freezing', myoclonic jerks, muscle spasms and/or muscle fasciculations. Behaviour disorders such as episodes of aggression or compulsive behaviour changes (stereotypic behaviours, e.g. continuous rhythmic pacing, licking and vocalisations) can also look similar to sensory seizures. Dogs and cats are usually normal in between episodes. Compulsive behaviour changes, however, are not associated with changes in muscle tone or in the level of consciousness, and usually, a behavioural trigger can be identified.

Vestibular attacks

Transient vestibular episodes are a rare phenomenon characterised by the same cardinal signs seen with non-intermittent vestibular disease such as head tilt, nystagmus and ataxia. Nystagmus and gait abnormalities can also be seen with seizures, but it is rare that a seizure causes a head tilt. These patients will typically have no altered consciousness during an episode and are fairly normal before and after an episode. These episodes will not respond to standard anti-epileptic drug treatment.

Paroxysmal movement disorders

Our understanding and therefore our ability to identify paroxysmal movement disorders have improved in the last decade. Most of the movement disorders are elicited or deteriorate when the animal is excited or gets stressed. They usually are associated with movements, rarely occur at rest or out of sleep, are episodic and involve an increase in muscle tone (dystonia) and do not affect the level of consciousness. Some of these paroxysmal movement disorders were formerly thought to be seizures, but they lacked adequate response to standard anti-epileptic drugs. In addition, they more closely resemble movement conditions described in humans, and so they are now considered to be a movement disorder. Some of them have been genetically characterised.

Table 7.1 Clinical characteristics of episodic disorders.

Discriminator	Syncope	Narcolepsy/cataplexy	Neuro-muscular weakness	Paroxysmal behaviour changes (compulsive disorder)	Vestibular attack	Paroxysmal dyskinesia	Idiopathic head tremor	Seizure
Between episodes	–	Altered sleep/wake cycle	–/show signs of weakness	–	–	–	–	– (idiopathic epilepsy)/abormal (structural epilepsy, reactive seizures)
Precipitating event/tTrigger	Exercise, excitement	Excitement, food, phar-macologically	Exercise, excitement	Behavioural triggers (e.g. fear)	–	–/movement or exercise	–	–/flashing lights
Pre-event changes	–	–	–	–	–	–	–	pre-ictal behaviour changes (prodrome [hours to days] and/or aura [minutes]) such as starring, freezing, attention seeking, fear
Event Description	Brief, sudden collapse and recovery	Sudden collapse	Stiff, stilted gait prior to collapse	For example, pacing, barking, licking, chasing imaginary objects, chewing objects	Head tilt, nystagmus, collapse/fall towards side of head tilt	Dystonia, ballismus, chorea, tremor, collapse	Tremor of head in 'Yes'/'No' direction	Depending on seizure focus, focal or generalized tonic-clonic movements most common

Table 7.1 (*continued*)

Discriminator	Syncope	Narcolepsy/ cataplexy	Neuro-muscular weakness	Paroxysmal behaviour changes (compulsive disorder)	Vestibular attack	Paroxysmal dyskinesia	Idiopathic head tremor	Seizure
Level of consciousness	Unconscious	Asleep	–	–	–/impaired (disorientated)	–	–	Impaired /unconscious
Autonomic signs	Heart rate/ rhythm changes possible	–	–	–	–	–	–	Hypersalivation, Defaecation, Urination
Muscle tone	Flaccid	Flaccid	– to flaccid	–	Unilateral decrease in extensor muscle tone	Hypertonicity	–	Tonic (hypertonicity)/ tonic-clonic alternating movement (convulsions)
Lateralising signs	–	–	–	–	Yes	Possible	–	Asymmetrical seizures (structural epilepsy)
Duration	Seconds	Seconds to minutes	Minutes to hours	Minutes to hours	Seconds to hours	Minutes	Minutes to hours	Seconds to minutes/ status epilepticus (>10 minutes)
Post-episodic changes	–	–	–	–	–	Can appear tired	–	Yes, such as behaviour changes, blindness, gait abnormalities
Further comments	–	–	–	–	Subtle signs of vestibular disease might persist	–	Episodes can stop when interrupted	Head/facial muscles often involved

'–' = normal, none or not shown

Neuromuscular weakness and syncope (see Chapter 6 for further details)

Canine epileptoide cramping syndrome

Canine epileptoide cramping syndrome ('Spike's disease') in Border Terriers is one of these examples. These episodes were formerly considered to be focal seizures, but they are now considered to be a sub-type of paroxysmal dyskinesias reported in people (paroxysmal dystonic choreoathetosis). Paroxysmal dyskinesias have been classified on the basis of phenomenology, duration of the events and precipitating factors. This last classification includes paroxysmal kinesigenic dyskinesia, if the attacks occur abruptly after a sudden voluntary movement; paroxysmal non-kinesigenic dyskinesia, if the attacks occur spontaneously; paroxysmal exertion-induced dyskinesia, if the attacks are precipitated by prolonged physical exertion and paroxysmal hypnogenic dyskinesia, if the episodes of involuntary movements occur only during sleep. Differentiating epileptic seizures from paroxysmal dyskinesia is also challenging in people. Paroxysmal dyskinesias are distinguishable from focal seizures by the lack of secondary generalisation of motor activity as would be seen in a generalised motor seizure. However, the muscle tone is often increased on both sides of the body (e.g. extended and increased muscle tone in two or four limbs), but the consciousness is not impaired as it would be if this would be a seizure affecting both brain hemispheres. Border Terriers affected by the syndrome have episodic mild tremors, dystonia and difficulties walking.

Chinook paroxysmal dyskinesia

A similar condition has been described in the Chinook dog. 'Chinook paroxysmal dyskinesia' episodes are characterised by dystonia (e.g. involuntary sustained muscle contractions causing twisted postures or repetitive movements), chorea (e.g. rapid, involuntary, non-stereotypical, semi- or non-purposeful movements of an extremity or extremities) and ballismus (e.g. violent, involuntary, non-stereotypical, rapid movement of an extremity or extremities). However, athetotic movements (slow, involuntary, non-stereotypical, non-purposeful movements of an extremity or extremities) have not been reported in these dogs. Autonomic signs are absent such as urination, defaecation and hypersalivation. The duration of episodes can range from minutes to an hour. The episodes are not triggered by sudden movement, and the animals are normal before and after an episode. However, after the episodes, dogs can appear tired, most likely because of the prolonged sustained increased muscle activity.

Episodic falling

Episodic falling in Cavalier King Charles Spaniel is an example of a paroxysmal exertion-induced dyskinesia, which is typically aggravated or induced by stress, excitement or exercise. It is characterised by episodes of increased muscle tone (muscular hypertonicity) of the limbs. These dogs appear not to be able to relax the affected muscles and can have a 'deer-stalking' gait. The back can become arched, and the head lowers to the ground before the dog falls over. These dogs appear normal following an episode and have a normal mentation during an episode. The episodes last from seconds to minutes. Concurrent autonomic signs have not been reported in this disorder.

Idiopathic head tremor

Movement disorders can affect specific body parts such as the head in idiopathic head tremors ('head bobbing'), which are described in dogs such as the Doberman Pinscher, Bulldog or Boxer. The head tremor has usually a frequency of 5/s, can be vertical and/or horizontal in direction, lasts seconds to hours, can occur multiple times per day, be triggered by certain positioning of the head and can be aggravated by stress or excitement. The tremors can be stopped or reduced when the animal is distracted, for example food. No autonomic signs have been described, and the animal has appropriate mentation during an episode.

Summary

As a rule of thumb, if you are presented with a purebred dog, which has a paroxysmal episode that does not cause autonomic dysfunction, is normal after the episode, does not look similar to a generalised tonic-clonic seizure, has appropriate mentation during an episode even if changes in muscle activity are bilateral and/or does not respond as well to anti-epileptic drugs, you should consult the relevant internet databases for a breed-specific movement disorder.

In brief, these paroxysmal movement disorders usually lack the following:

- an identifiable precipitating event such as an aura (sensory seizure activity, such as behaviour change [attention seeking, sniffing and starring], lasting a couple of minutes just before the motor seizure activity)
- autonomic signs (e.g. hypersalivation, urination and defaecation)
- generalisation of increased motor activity (e.g. generalised tonic or tonic-clonic seizure)
- an impairment of consciousness. Usually, dogs with impaired consciousness will not be able to look into the owner's eyes during the event, and this is a good question to ask the owner. Animals will also often not listen to the owner due to the impairment of consciousness, although this is often falsely under-reported due to the owner's perception of the event.

Seizures

The brain is a 'complex' structure but has only 'simple' (limited) ways of expressing dysfunction. A seizure is a clinical sign caused by forebrain dysfunction – it is not a diagnosis (one specific disease). A plethora of structural and functional causes can result in seizures (see the following section when we talk about defining the lesion). Seizures can have many forms depending on which part of the brain is affected by seizure generation and propagation; for example, a seizure could just affect a specific part of the sensory cortex and the animal might only have a change in behaviour (starring, freezing, sniffing, etc.) or only one part of the motor cortex is affected and the animal only demonstrates orofacial automatisms. The location of the 'symptomatogenic' zone (area of the brain causing the observed clinical signs) usually overlays or is close to the epileptogenic zone (area of the brain causing the seizure) and therefore indicates the origin of the seizure. Seizure semiology, using clinical signs of cerebral dysfunctions caused by a seizure, not only helps to confirm that the event is a seizure, but also provides information about its origin. It is relatively simple and is clinically cost effective. Depending on the brain areas or parts being affected by the seizure motor, sensory (including behaviour changes) and vegetative changes and automatisms can be differentiated and help to characterise the seizure event.

Is it a seizure?

In brief:

- Increased muscle tone is far more likely in seizures. The most common recognised seizure is a generalised tonic-clonic seizure. Most commonly, the animal first goes stiff (tonic phase), loses proprioception and collapses into lateral recumbency, then the tonic-clonic phase (rhythmic alternating muscle contractions) starts, followed often by running movements (automatisms). Atonic seizures are very uncommon, and a 'floppy' collapse should guide the clinician to 'think' syncope or cataplexy.
- Rhythmic alternating muscle contractions are common in both focal and generalised seizures.
- Seizures often first involve the head and facial muscles (eye or facial muscle twitching).
- Stereotypical – most animals will have only one (or two) type(s) of seizure (seizure onset generalized, focal seizure onset with or without secondary generalisation). Seizures in an animal typically originate from the same epileptic focus and spread following the same brain pathways.
- The ictus (seizure itself) normally lasts 1–2 minutes.
- Most seizures exhibit several stages:
  - pre-ictal behaviour changes (prodrome [hours to days] and/or aura [minutes])
  - ictus
  - post-ictal behaviour or neurological deficits (hours to days).

Apart from the seizure itself, it is the post-ictal changes that are recognised by the owner.

- Common post-ictal dysfunctions are as follows:
  - behaviour changes such as fear, aggression and disorientation
  - increased appetite
  - compulsive pacing
  - blindness, usually with normal pupillary light reflexes consistent with 'central' blindness
  - menace response deficits
  - miosis contralateral to the lesion (if one lesion [secondary to disinhibition of the oculomotor nucleus])
  - gait abnormalities, especially ataxia and 'conscious' proprioceptive (paw position) deficits

- Seizures often, but not always, occur at rest or while sleeping.
- Seizures usually impair the consciousness of the animal.
- Most of the seizure disorders will at least initially respond to anti-epileptic treatment.

2 Define the system

Defining the problem appropriately is essential for paroxysmal disorders, as the different problems will guide you to rank the systems involved in order of priority. If the presenting complaint is a seizure(s), a vestibular episode, cataplectic attacks, episodic behaviour changes or a movement disorder, the system that needs to be examined more closely is the central nervous system (CNS). It can be affected either directly or indirectly. In addition to causing changes in behaviour, seizures or movement disorders will have an effect on the neuromuscular system, but this would be 'ranked' below the CNS in importance. Vestibular disorder can be caused by CNS and peripheral nervous system dysfunction, and a brief discussion of how this occurs can be found in the following section. Other conditions discussed previously (syncope and neuromuscular weakness) also affect the neuromuscular system. A discussion of which other systems might be involved in these clinical presentations and how they can be prioritised can be found in Chapter 6.

3 Define the location

Once you have established that the peripheral or CNS is involved, the neurological examination can assist you to localise the lesion to an exact neuroanatomical location. Despite recent developments in advanced imaging, the neurological examination is still the key to open the drawer to gain access to the most appropriate diagnostics to help you identify the underlying cause of the condition. Especially with seizure disorders, it can be helpful to determine if the lesion is located peripherally (extra-cranial) or centrally (intra-cranial), as this can guide the diagnostic pathway to efficiently establish a diagnosis.

Vestibular attacks

An appreciation of the vestibular system's function is important to help you understand how to localise the lesion correctly and why this is important. The vestibular system's main function is to maintain an animal's equilibrium during movement and orientation against gravity. It is divided into two main sections: the *peripheral* ('extra-axial', peripheral to brainstem and cerebellum) and the *central* ('intra-axial', within brainstem) part. The sensory receptors of the vestibular system are located in the inner ear (petrosal bone). The information recorded by the sensory receptors is transmitted via the peripheral cranial nerve VIII (CNVIII; vestibulocochlear nerve) to the vestibular nuclei located in the brainstem just below the cerebellum. Some of the nerve fibres continue their path and also communicate to a part of the cerebellum. The peripheral system detects linear acceleration and rotational movement of the head.

The vestibular system is responsible for maintaining the position of the eyes, neck, trunk and limbs with reference to the position of the head. The vestibular nuclei communicate with the nuclei of the nerves controlling eye positioning and movement. Other pathways connect the vestibular nuclei with the cerebellum, cerebrum, other brainstem centre (e.g. vomiting centre; Chapter 2) and the spinal cord.

The vestibular system is a *unilateral* system, which means that the left vestibular system controls the posture of the left side of the animal, and the right one controls the right side. The vestibular nuclei give rise mainly to a pathway that is facilitatory to extensor muscles. However, some fibres inhibit contralateral extensor tone and ipsilateral flexor muscles. Keeping this in mind, it is logical that a head tilt and a reduced extensor tone of the limbs are towards or on the side of the lesion. 'It looks like the animal is running around a curve'. The jerk nystagmus develops from the dysfunction of the pathways connecting the vestibular nuclei with the cranial nerve nuclei responsible for the eye movement. The slow phase of the jerk nystagmus goes into the direction of the lesion; the fast phase is the compensatory one. Vision and proprioception can help to compensate for vestibular dysfunction. Vestibular disease can progressively improve, as other parts of the brain can 'override' some of the lack of sensory vestibular input, but clinical signs deteriorate when the animal is blinded.

Clinical signs of dysfunction of the vestibular system are as follows:

1 loss of balance
2 head tilt

3 leaning towards one side
4 rolling
5 circling
6 jerk nystagmus
7 positional strabismus
8 and depending on the type of vestibular disease (central vs. 'peripheral'), other cranial nerve deficits, Horner's Syndrome, cerebellar signs, mental depression and hemiparesis with postural reaction deficits can be observed.

By defining the clinical signs present, you will be able to distinguish central vs. 'peripheral' vestibular disease, and this will direct you to focus your workup on intra-cranial vs. extra-cranial disease (Figure 7.1).

If you have brainstem dysfunction including vestibular signs, then think 'central vestibular'. If you have a head tilt away from the side of postural reaction deficits, then think 'paradoxical vestibular' (cerebellum or cerebellomedullary pontine angle). If you have *no* signs of brainstem involvement, then think 'peripheral vestibular' (if facial nerve deficits and/or Horner's syndrome in addition to peripheral vestibular disease, consider tympanic bulla disorders).

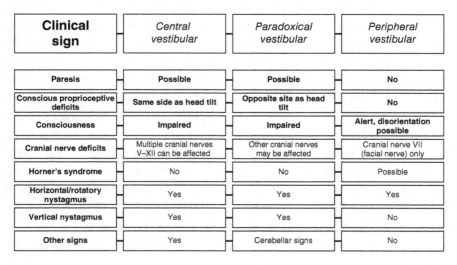

Clinical sign	*Central vestibular*	*Paradoxical vestibular*	*Peripheral vestibular*
Paresis	**Possible**	**Possible**	**No**
Conscious proprioceptive deficits	**Same side as head tilt**	**Opposite site as head tilt**	**No**
Consciousness	**Impaired**	**Impaired**	**Alert, disorientation possible**
Cranial nerve deficits	Multiple cranial nerves V–XII can be affected	Other cranial nerves may be affected	Cranial nerve VII (facial nerve) only
Horner's syndrome	No	No	Possible
Horizontal/rotatory nystagmus	Yes	Yes	Yes
Vertical nystagmus	Yes	Yes	No
Other signs	Yes	Cerebellar signs	No

Figure 7.1 The combination of clinical signs determines the location of the lesion.

The head tilt is to the side ipsilateral to the lesion, unless, the lesion is in the flocculonodular lobe of the cerebellum or the cerebellomedullary pontine angle, then the patient may have a paradoxical head tilt. In this case, the head tilts to the contralateral side. Because the lesion involves the cerebellar projections to the vestibular nuclei, and because the cerebellum is predominantly inhibitory in effect, the side of the lesion becomes overactive, giving excessive tone to the extensors of that side and causing the patient to lean and tilt away from the lesion. However, the side of the lesion can be determined by testing the proprioception, especially paw positioning, which is reduced to absent on the side of the lesion.

Sometimes, the patient may present with bilateral vestibular disease. One typically sees wide excursions of the head ('Stevie Wonder head movement'), symmetrical ataxia and no head tilt, and the patient may not demonstrate a 'normal' physiological nystagmus. Bilateral vestibular diseases are usually peripheral in location. Metronidazole intoxication and thiamine deficiency are the exception, which can cause bilateral central vestibular disease.

Narcolepsy, paroxysmal behaviour changes and paroxysmal movement disorders

The most important step in defining the location for these disorders is identification of the episode you are dealing with. These disorders are caused by a brain dysfunction – either by an intra-cranial or by an extra-cranial cause. If you find on your neurological examination signs of lateralisation (asymmetrical neurological deficits) or skull/neck pain, then intra-cranial structural lesions are more likely (see the following sections for more detail).

Seizures

Seizures = forebrain dysfunction. Your neurological examination will therefore need to centre on assessing forebrain function. But do not ignore the rest of the neurological examination, as identification of multifocal or widespread neurological disease might alter your clinical reasoning.

Seizures themselves can be the first and the only initial sign of structural brain disease, such as neoplasia in the 'silent areas of the brain' (silent areas are those areas that cannot be examined by the neurological examination, e.g. frontal or olfactory lobe). However, more commonly, the neurological examination might identify the following neurological deficits in dogs with intra-cranial – *structural* fore *brain disease*:

- Mentation changes (quality – behaviour changes such as compulsive pacing, head pressing and head turn and/or level – obtundation)
- Postural reaction deficits (such as decreased or absent paw positioning) contralateral to the lesion and/or hemiparesis
- Vision deficits contralateral to the lesion
- Decreased or absent menace response, with normal pupillary light reflex contralateral to the lesion
- Reduced facial sensation and response to nasal septum stimulation contralateral to the lesion
- Ad addendum:
  - Some animals might have neurological deficits affecting both sides equally
  - Focal-onset asymmetrical seizures (seizures that affect one body side more than the other) can indicate structural brain lesion contralateral to the more affected body side (e.g. facial twitches on the left side indicate a right forebrain lesion).

Dogs and cats with seizures secondary to extra-cranial causes can have similar neurological deficits, but they are usually symmetrical in presentation. The clinical signs might be waxing and waning. The inter-ictal neurological examination can be normal for extra-cranial and functional intra-cranial causes, as seizures can be the only clinical sign of forebrain dysfunction. Post-ictal cerebral dysfunction can cause neurological deficits for hours to days. The clinician should therefore repeat the neurological examination, if neurological deficits are found in close proximity to the last seizure event.

4 Define the lesion

Vestibular attacks

The diagnostic workup may vary greatly between central vs. peripheral disease. Depending on the onset and clinical course, diseases can be grouped into acute onset, non-progressive or progressive and chronic progressive (Tables 7.2 and 7.3). Furthermore, thinking

Table 7.2 Potential differential diagnoses for 'peripheral' vestibular disease.

Category	Acute non-progressive	Acute progressive	Chronic progressive
Degenerative			Congenital vestibular syndrome (often also deaf)
Metabolic		Hypothyroidism (diabetes mellitus; indirect)	Hypothyroidism
Neoplastic		Metastatic	Soft tissue tumours Nerve sheath tumour
Inflammatory/ infectious		*Otitis media/interna (bacterial/fungal)* *Protozoal*	*Otitis media/interna (bacterial/fungal)* *Protozoal*
Idiopathic	Idiopathic	Sterile otitis media with effusion	Sterile otitis media with effusion
Traumatic	*Fracture*		
Toxic		Streptomycin Gentamycin	Streptomycin Gentamycin
Vascular	Infarction Haemorrhage		

Lesions that can be associated with pain are shown in italics

pathophysiologically, diseases that can be associated with pain are inflammatory, infectious or neoplastic conditions. Apart from checking for neck pain and palpating the skull and ear area, you can also check if the animal has pain opening its mouth.

An easy way to refine your lesion is to use what we have called a 'five-finger' rule:

1 Onset
2 Clinical course
3 Pain
4 Lateralisation (asymmetrical neurological deficits)
5 Neuroanatomical localisation.

The use of this five-finger rule can help you reduce your differential list, for example an animal with a chronic, progressive, painful, left-sided peripheral vestibular disease has most likely an inflammatory, infectious or neoplastic middle/inner ear condition. Given the

Table 7.3 Potential differential diagnoses for central vestibular disease.

Category	Acute non-progressive	Acute progressive	Chronic progressive
Anomalous			(*Hydrocephalus*)
Degenerative			Neurodegenerative diseases Storage diseases
Metabolic		Hypothyroidism	Hypothyroidism
Neoplastic		*Metastatic*	Primary: *Choroid plexus tumour*, glioma, meningioma, *lymphoma*
Nutritional		Thiamine deficiency (usually bilateral)	
Inflammatory/ infectious		*MUA* *FIP, canine distemper* *Protozoal, fungal*	*MUA* *FIP, canine distemper* *Protozoal, fungal*
Toxic		Lead Hexachlorophene Metronidazole (usually bilateral)	Lead Hexachlorophene
Traumatic	Fracture/bleed		
Vascular	Infarction Haemorrhage		

Lesions that can be associated with pain are shown in italics. (MUA = Meningoencephalomyelitis of Unknown Aetiology; FIP = Feline Infectious Peritonitis)

peripheral vestibular location, radiography of the skull with oblique views and open mouth can be considered (especially in cats), but the main investigation will be an otoscopic examination of the external ear canal and the tympanic membrane (Figure 7.2). If the potential for otitis media exists, then myringotomy is a diagnostic option, although it does require a general anaesthetic. Cultures (fungal and bacterial) and cytology should be obtained from within the bullae. Cytology, in particular, will allow differentiation of active infection from normal middle ear flora, bearing in mind that the middle ear communicates with the oral cavity via the eustachian tube. Take note that the tympanic bullae of the dog are anatomically different from

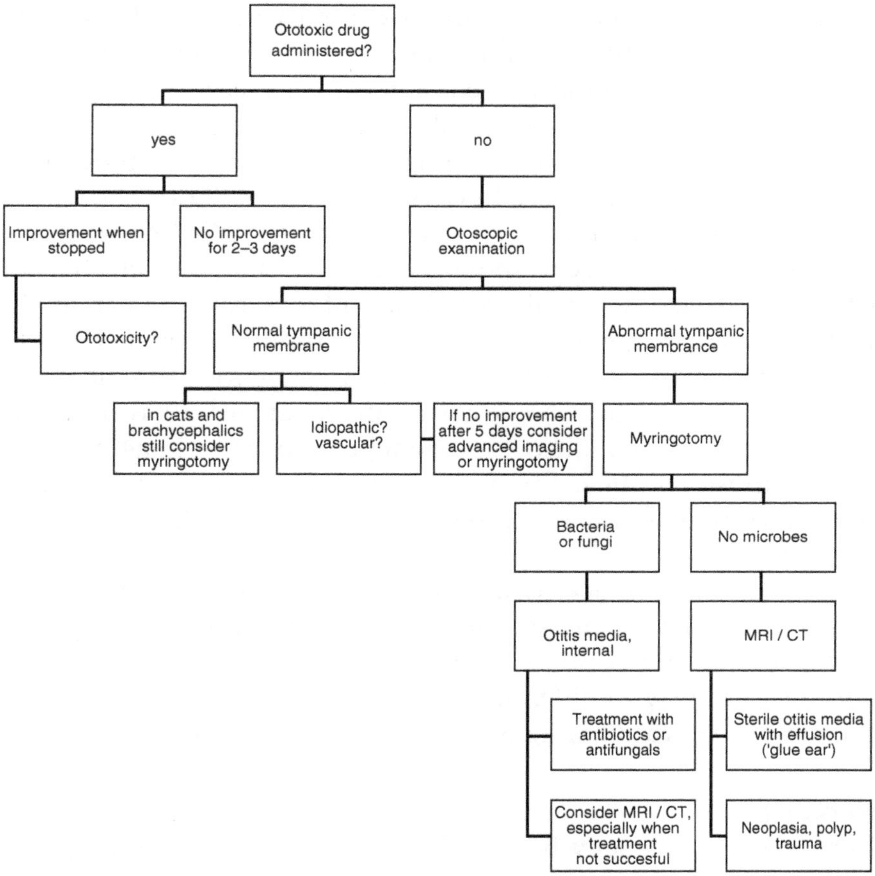

Figure 7.2 Algorithm for peripheral vestibular work-up.

those of the cat. The tympanic bulla of both species contains two compartments. In the cat, there is a near-closed membrane between the two, whereas in the dog, both compartments communicate with each other. Myringotomy should be performed in the ventrocaudal quadrant of the tympanic membrane where the resultant puncture in the membrane is quick to heal. Wound healing can be prolonged in patients treated with, for example systemic glucocorticoids, or systemic disease, such as diabetes mellitus.

The differentiation of the various central vestibular diseases will usually require advanced imaging (Table 7.3). This is the most important reason to localise the lesion correctly, as it will change the workup of the case. It is generally believed that lesion localisation has to do with determining the prognosis. However, the prognosis is determined by the diagnosed disease process, *not* by the location of the lesion. Animals have been diagnosed with soft tissue sarcomas invading the middle ear (poor prognosis), and conversely, dogs have been diagnosed with cerebellar infarcts causing paradoxical vestibular disease (good prognosis). Structural lesions affecting the brain parenchyma will not be seen with conventional radiography. These lesions may be mass lesions, infarcts or just areas of inflammation that will enhance on magnetic resonance imaging (MRI) with contrast. For the definitive diagnosis of inflammatory/infectious central vestibular disease, cerebrospinal fluid (CSF) evaluation is required.

The vestibular attack, which can be challenging to diagnose and be confused with seizure secondary to idiopathic epilepsy, might be a transient ischaemic vestibular attack. No pathology can be identified, and the only way to differentiate these episodes from seizures is by the presence of cardinal signs of vestibular dysfunction.

Narcolepsy

Narcolepsy can usually be identified by characterising the episode. If you are uncertain, you can trigger an episode by food and/or excitement or pharmacologically (e.g. physostigmine). Familial (e.g. Labrador Retriever and Doberman Pinscher) and sporadic forms have been described. Make sure that you ask if other animals in the litter or the breeding line have been affected. A gene test is available for the familial form, which is caused by a defect in the hypocretin receptor 2 gene. To identify the sporadic form, an intra-cranial workup (MRI and CSF analysis) is required. Special laboratories can measure CSF hypocretin levels, which might be reduced in the sporadic form. An extra-cranial workup needs to be considered (see the following section) if you are not completely confident that the 'strange' episode(s) observed can be explained by narcolepsy.

Table 7.4 Potential differential diagnoses for syncope.

Category	Differentials	Diagnostics
Syncope		
Cardiovascular	Left-sided heart failure	Thoracic radiographs, echocardiography
	Paroxysmal arrhythmias	Electrocardiography, echocardiography
	Heartworm disease	Thoracic radiographs, Baermann, antigen detection
	Severe anaemia	Haematology (and see Chapter 9)
	Hyperviscosity syndromes	Haematology, serum biochemistry
Respiratory	Severe upper airways disease	Haematology, endoscopy, radiographs/CT
Metabolic	Hypoglycaemia	(Fasten) blood glucose

Syncope

Your physical examination findings will guide your workup. Depending on the clinical signs and the system you have identified, following differentials need to be considered (Table 7.4).

Paroxysmal behaviour changes

It can be difficult sometimes to differentiate paroxysmal behavioural changes from seizures that mainly affect the behaviour of an animal. If you are uncertain whether the episode could be a seizure, then follow the workup scheme presented as follows for seizure disorders.

Paroxysmal movement disorders

Currently, we have only very limited availability to characterise these *paroxysmal movement disorders*. Genetics has improved our understanding of these disorders and will continue to do so. It is therefore recommended to search the Internet when you suspect an episode to be a movement disorder; for example, a gene defect in *BCAN* has been *identified for* episodic falling in Cavalier King Charles Spaniel and a gene test is available.

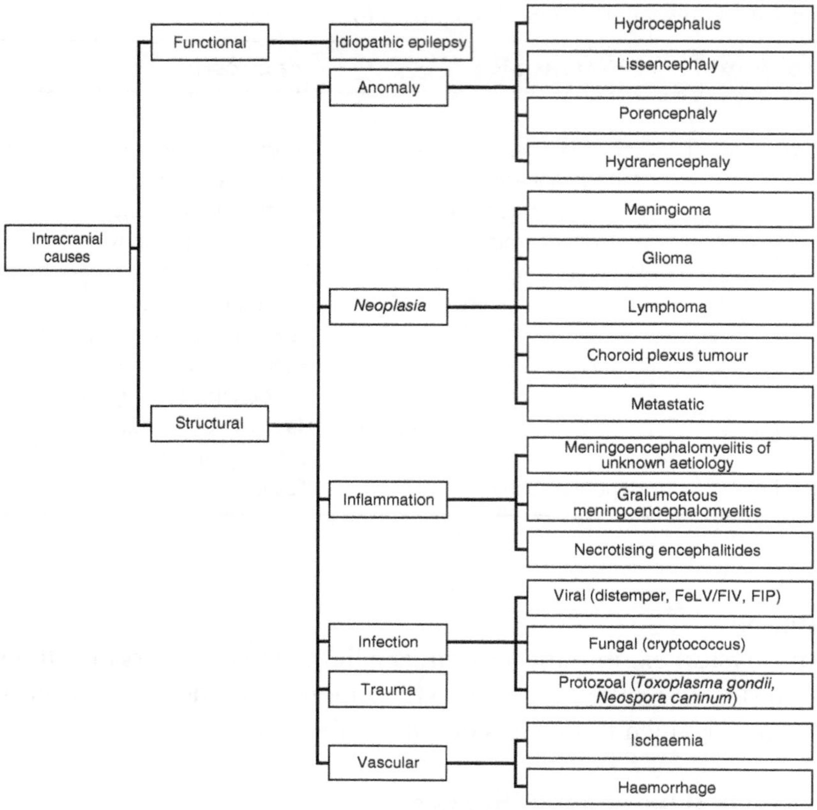

Figure 7.3 Intracranial causes for seizures.

Seizures

Extra-cranial vs. intra-cranial

Seizures are caused by either extra-cranial or intra-cranial diseases, which alter cerebral function (Figures 7.3–7.5; Tables 7.5 and 7.6).

Intra-cranial causes

Intra-cranial causes can be further subdivided into the following:

- Functional disorders
  - Idiopathic or primary epilepsy (a genetic component is suspected)
  - No visible structural changes of the brain on MRI or gross pathological examination
  - Unremarkable inter-ictal neurological examination

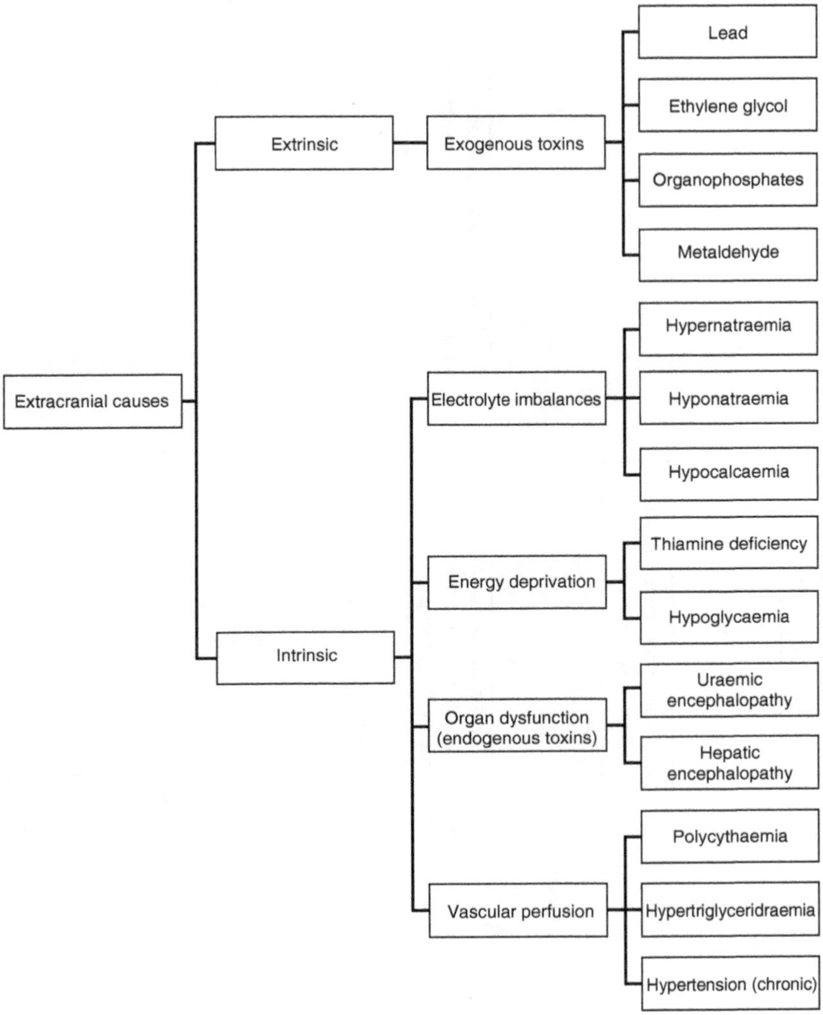

Figure 7.4 Extracranial causes for (reactive) seizure.

- Structural diseases
  - Structural epilepsy
  - Presence of gross structural changes of the brain causing asymmetrical neurological deficits or seizures, for example neoplasms, inflammatory/infectious causes, vascular accidents and cerebral anomalies.

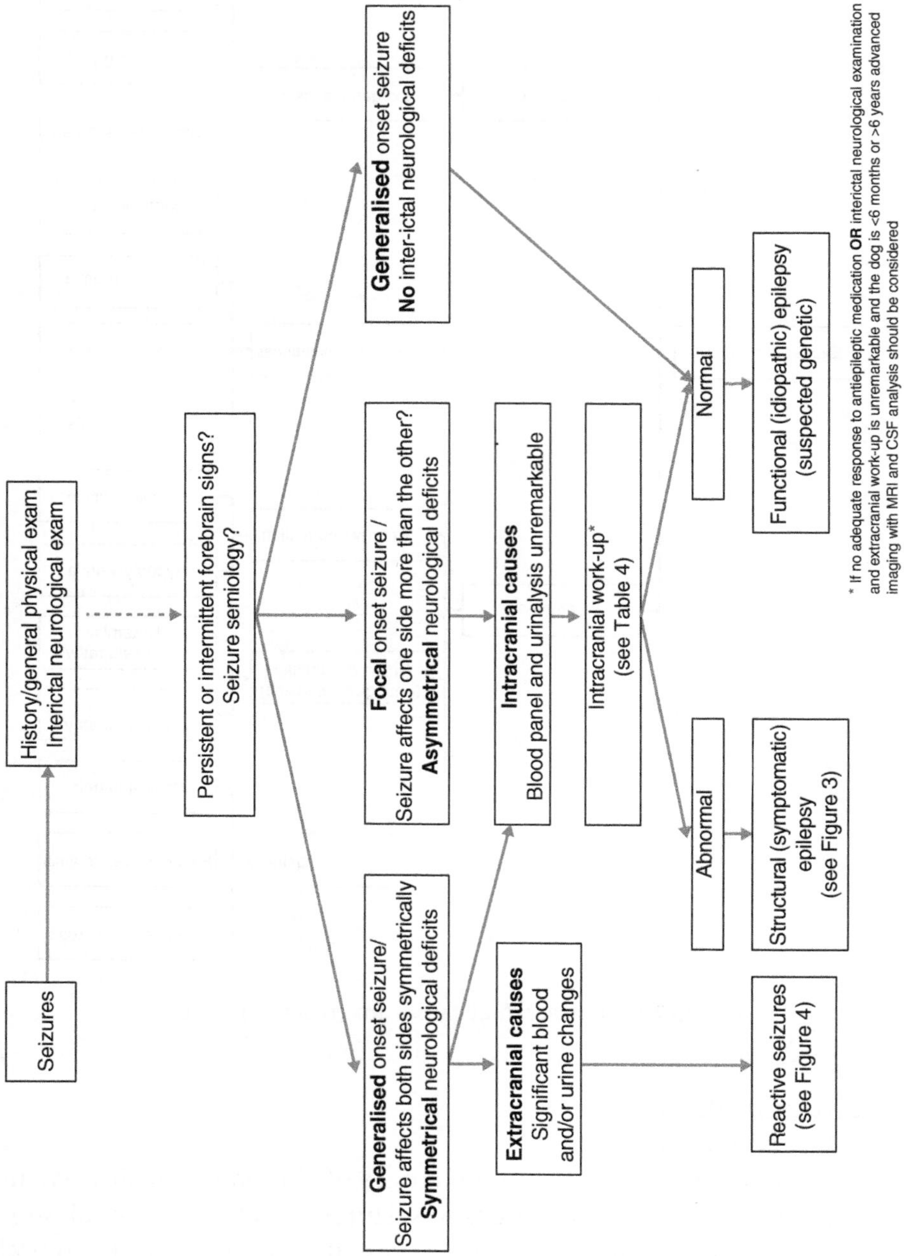

Figure 7.5 Flow chart to help define the lesion.

Table 7.5 Diagnostic tests to consider for dogs and cats presenting with seizures.

Extracranial	Intracranial

• Haematology
• Serum biochemical profile
• Pre- and postprandial bile acids
• Ammonium biurate crystals (urine)/ Ammonia (blood)
• Urinalysis
• Blood pressure/ Fundus examination
• Serology/PCR e.g. *Toxoplasma gondii*, *Neospora caninum*, canine distemper, FeLV/FIV, FIP, Cryptococcus
• Genetic characterisation e.g. *Epm2b*, *LGI2,* L2-hydroxyglutaric aciduria, neuronal ceroid lipofuscinosis
• Serum lead concentration
	• Advanced imaging
	  ○ MRI
	  ○ CT
	• Cerebrospinal fluid analysis
	  ○ Cytology
	  ○ Protein
	  ○ PCR (*Toxoplasma gondii, Neospora caninum*, canine distemper virus, FeCoV)
	• Electroencephalogram

- ○ Intra-cranial disease cannot be ruled out completely if the animal is completely normal between seizures
- ○ Usually, these dogs will not respond adequately to anti-epileptic treatment.
- ○ Structural lesions that are too small to cause neurological dysfunction other than seizures or are in a relatively 'silent' area of the forebrain may not manifest in any way other than seizures.

We have shown that finding asymmetrical neurological deficits on the inter-ictal neurological examination increases significantly (by 25 times) the likelihood of finding intra-cranial structural brain disease. Finding symmetrical deficits, cluster seizures and focal-onset (usually asymmetrical) seizures also significantly increases the chance of finding intra-cranial pathology. If you then take age and breed into account, you can refine your differential list substantially. The neurological examination is a powerful tool! Some animals might have other neurological deficits unrelated to the seizure disorder (e.g. chronic lumbosacral disease), so always make sure you take a holistic view on the case.

Table 7.6 Neurological examination findings, seizure semiology and signalment can help to create a list of differential diagnoses.

	Inter-ictal neurological examination			Seizure type		Age			
Differentials	**Normal**	**Symmetrical abnormal**	**Asymmetrical abnormal**	**Symmetrical generalised onset**	**Asymmetrical – focal onset***	**<6 months**	**6 months – 6 years**	**>6 years**	**Breed**
Degenerative		X		X				X	X
Focal anomalies			X		X	X			
Hydrocephalus		X		X		X			
Metabolic (e.g. portosystemic shunt)	(X)	X		X		X	(X)		
Neoplasia			*X*		*X*		*(X)*	*X*	*(X)*
Midline neoplasia (e.g. pituitary tumour)		X		X			(X)	X	(X)
Nutritional		X		X		X	X	X	
Inflammation/ infection			*X*		*X*		*X*	*(X)*	*(X)*
Idiopathic epilepsy	X			X			X	X^	X
Toxin	(X)	X		X		X	X	X	
Trauma			X		X	X	X	X	
Vascular			X		X			X	

*Focal seizure can secondary generalise – focus on seizure onset; ^Late-onset; *Lesions which can be associated with pain are shown in italics*

Generalised onset (symmetrical) seizures are more common with idiopathic epilepsy, metabolic, toxic and degenerative causes and with hydrocephalus. Since metabolic and toxic disease tends to have diffuse, symmetrical effects on the brain, seizures tend to be generalized and symmetrical in onset. The lack of inter-ictal neurological deficits and clinical examination findings are the most important predictors for the diagnosis of idiopathic epilepsy. If you also consider breed (especially familial history of seizures) and the age of onset (6 months–6 years), you have more than a 95% chance that idiopathic epilepsy is the cause of the seizure disorder.

Many breeds are predisposed to have epilepsy. A hereditary and familial basis for idiopathic epilepsy has been proposed in a number of breeds, including the Golden Retriever, Labrador Retriever, Australian-, German- and Belgian Shepherd (Tervueren), Bernese Mountain dog, Beagle, Irish wolfhound, English Springer Spaniel, Keeshond, Hungarian Vizsla, Standard Poodle, Border Collie and Lagotto Romagnolo. There is currently only a gene test for the Lagotto Romagnolo and Belgian Tervueren for idiopathic (genetic) epilepsy.

Extra-cranial causes

Extra-cranial causes can impair the function of the CNS and cause *reactive seizures*. The seizures will stop when the metabolic or toxic cause is rectified. For example:

- reduced delivery of nutrients to the brain
  - for example glucose and thiamine
- impairment of vascular function
  - for example hyperviscosity syndrome (hypertriglyceridaemia and polycythaemia) and hypertension
- changes in the internal milieu of neurons that alter their function
  - for example calcium and sodium imbalances
- exposure to extrinsic or intrinsic toxins
  - for example metaldehyde and portosystemic shunt.

The lesion can be further defined by considering the history and clinical examination findings. Observations more commonly reported in seizures caused by extra-cranial metabolic disease include the following:

- waxing and waning clinical signs (often involving the level of mentation)

- chronological association of clinical signs to feeding
- gastrointestinal disturbances
- increased or decreased appetite
- pica
- hypersalivation.

Extra-cranial disease may or may not cause clinical signs in addition to seizures. Metabolic disturbances such as hyperkalaemia due to hypoadrenocorticism and hypocalcaemia most commonly will also cause signs of malaise, such as gastrointestinal dysfunction, but there are occasional reports of dogs with these disorders where seizures were the only presenting sign. Hypoglycaemia will frequently cause seizures with no other clinical signs. Confirmation of hypoglycaemia may be problematical, as homeostatic mechanisms (adrenaline and cortisol release) will come into play when the blood glucose falls to a critical level and increase the blood glucose temporarily. It is important to obtain a fasting blood glucose sample when investigating metabolic causes of seizures.

The clinician should also always ensure that they ask the owners if exposure to a toxin is possible. Only a few toxins can be easily identified on blood work analysis, and there are few laboratories available that can analyse samples for toxins and provide guidance for companion animals. Good history taking is therefore essential. The most commonly reported toxins causing seizures are lead, ethylene glycol, organophosphates and metaldehyde.

Most of the diagnostics for extra-cranial causes of seizures (metabolic or toxic) can be performed in first opinion practice (detailed history, blood and urine tests, blood pressure measurements, examination of the retina [convoluted and/or dilated blood vessels, bleeding] for signs of hypertension and imaging modalities accessible in first opinion practice such as ultrasonography; Table 7.5). The suspicion of an intra-cranial lesion usually requires advanced imaging techniques (computer tomography [CT] or ideally MRI) and CSF analysis to help differentiate the various aetiologies. Hydrocephalus can often be diagnosed with a brain ultrasound through an open fontanelle (common in animals affected with a congenital hydrocephalus). Most infectious diseases can be tested for by serology or PCR.

Some breeds have a predisposition, genetic susceptibility or causative mutation for diseases which are or can be associated with seizures. Examples include

- mutation in *Epm2b* causing Lafora body storage disease and progressive myoclonic epilepsy described in wire-haired Dachshounds, Beagles and Basset Hounds
- L2-hydroxyglutaric aciduria in Staffordshire Bull Terriers
- neuronal ceroid lipofuscinosis in Border Collie, English Setter, Australian Shepherd, American Bulldog, Dachshound, American Staffordshire and Tibetan Terrier
- Gliomas in Boxers
- Meningoencephalomyelitis of unknown aetiology in certain Terrier breeds.

In conclusion

Syncope, narcolepsy/cataplexy, pain, compulsive behaviour disorders, vestibular attacks, certain movement disorders, neuromuscular weakness and seizures are paroxysmal events, which share some commonalities in clinical presentation, but using a stepwise approach, you will not only be able to differentiate these episodes, but also be able to determine the most likely diagnosis.

CHAPTER 8

Sneezing, dyspnoea, coughing and other respiratory signs

David B. Church
The Royal Veterinary College, London, UK

This chapter deals with a logical approach to a group of signs that can be attributed to disturbances in the function of the respiratory tract.

1 Define the problem

Clinical signs referable to the respiratory tract are usually obvious and not easily confused with other clinical signs. There are a few exceptions however. Gagging after coughing is sometimes interpreted by owners as indicating that the major problem is vomiting (see Chapter 2) and will present their pet to the veterinarian for this problem.

The assessment of respiratory signs, however, can often be refined by defining the problem in greater detail. For example, sneezing generally is associated with nasal discharge – what is its character? Is the dyspnoea in a patient associated with coughing, or is there minimal, if any, coughing present? Is this animal presented for coughing dyspnoeic as well, or is there minimal evidence for dyspnoea? By considering these questions and thus attempting to more precisely define the problem, we can construct a logical approach to investigating disorders that predominantly affect the respiratory tract, which will facilitate more accurate explanations and effective management of the disorders encountered.

2 Define the system

When the clinician is faced with a presenting problem of sneezing, nasal discharge, coughing, dyspnoea and haemoptysis, the answer to

Clinical Reasoning in Small Animal Practice, First Edition.
Jill E. Maddison, Holger A. Volk and David B. Church.

the question 'what system is involved?' is clearly – the respiratory system.

Diseases that alter respiratory function may be *primary* problems of the respiratory tract (e.g. nasal neoplasia), they may be *primary* respiratory problems caused by severe dysfunction of another body system (e.g. pulmonary oedema due to severe left-sided heart failure) or they may be *secondary* to a disease that produces derangements, which alter respiratory function *without directly affecting* the respiratory system (e.g. tachypnoea or dyspnoea in a severely anaemic animal).

Sneezing and nasal discharge

2 Define the location

Sneezing and nasal discharge are typically signs of disease affecting the nasal cavity, the nasal sinuses, the cranial oropharynx and the dental arcade. On rare occasions when a disorder is both erosive and sufficiently well established, lesions of the hard palate may also result in nasal discharge and sneezing.

Clinical signs

The clinical signs of nasal disease are principally excessive snorting or sneezing with nasal discharge that may have varying consistencies, contain various amounts of blood (epistaxis) and be either unilateral or bilateral. Ulceration or excoriation of the nares, discharging sinuses from the maxillary bones forming the lateral walls of the nasal cavity or irritation of parts of the nasal cavity are uncommon findings but generally significant when present. Less commonly, distortions of the bones surrounding or adjacent to the nasal cavity may be detected as may increased prominence of one or both ocular globes.

All of the above-mentioned signs are highly suggestive of primary and thus structural nasal disease. In small animals, occasionally, epistaxis may reflect a systemic coagulopathy. However, usually the clinician's index of suspicion for a systemic problem resulting in secondary respiratory tract involvement is alerted by the presence of accompanying signs in other body systems and the absence of other signs referable to the respiratory tract.

Patients with primary nasal disease generally do not cough or wheeze. Dogs will also not have significant dyspnoea unless forced to breathe through their nose as occurs when they sleep in positions that result in their mouth being closed. While their nasal cavity may be totally occluded with no air movement evident at the external nares, this will not result in dyspnoea unless their mouth is forced closed, as they will accommodate readily by breathing through their open mouth.

Cats seem to be far less comfortable in breathing through their mouth, hence nasal cavity obstruction in the cat may also result in degrees of dyspnoea, although when the nasal disease is this severe, the clinical picture is generally dominated by the discharge and sneezing, which focuses attention on the nasal cavity as the part of the respiratory tract primarily affected.

Diagnostic aids

Patients with structural nasal discharge are likely to require the following diagnostic procedures:

- Imaging of the nasal cavity, sinuses and oropharynx. Diagnostic precision is substantially enhanced if CT imaging can be used, although if not available, standard radiological views can be helpful in many cases
- Rhinoscopy – both antegrade and retrograde views are essential
- Nasal biopsies.

In view of the invasive nature of these procedures and/or the need for significant immobilisation, it is most practical to perform all of the procedures at one time, avoiding multiple anaesthetics.

In certain situations, other diagnostic aids might be worth considering. Chief amongst these is serology to determine the level of crypotococcal antigen in patients where nasal cryptococossis is suspected. In general, the use of nasal washings and standard bacterial cultures is of little, if any, value, as primary bacterial inflammation of the nasal cavity is almost never encountered.

4 Define the lesion

Nasal pathology is due to either inflammation (infectious or non-infectious), neoplasia or malformations.

Inflammatory – infectious

Primary nasal disease versus systemic infectious disease with a nasal component

Nasal discharge may occur as part of a systemic infection, for example calicivirus or herpes infection in cats, or it may occur due to primary nasal disease. If due to primary nasal disease, it is important to ascertain if the problem is acute or chronic, as many acute problems resolve with minimal therapy.

If the problem is a chronic purulent discharge, then it is due to bacterial infection secondary to disruption of the normal balance between the bacteria colonising the nasal cavity as commensals and the mucosal barrier. Primary bacterial rhinitis without an underlying cause, rarely if ever occurs in cats or dogs. The usual explanations are neoplasia, a foreign body, a fungal infection or a tooth root abscess that has become continuous with the maxillary sinus and thus the nasal cavity or the nasal cavity itself.

Mycotic rhinitides

Mycotic rhinitides are generally caused by infections with organisms from the geni *Cryptococcus, Aspergillus* or *Penicillium*. Cryptococcal infections are more common in cats, while Aspergillosis is typically a problem in the dog.

Cryptococcosis

Cryptococcosis is an important but relatively uncommon disease of cats throughout the world. The disease is generally caused by infection with *Cryptococcus neoformans*, an encapsulated yeast with two biotypes, *C. neoformans* var *neoformans* and *C. neoformans* var *gattii*.

Isolates can vary within geographical regions. For example, in Australia, *C. neoformans* var *neoformans* is the more common isolate from cats in NSW, while the distribution of *C. neoformans* var *gattii* appears to be associated with pollen dispersal from river red gums (*Eucalyptus camaldulensis*), which are more commonly found in the more southern and western regions of the country.

Infection usually involves the nasal cavity. Skin, subcutis and the central nervous system have been implicated as common sites for infection. However, the vast majority of animals with cryptococcosis have nasal disease as the predominant clinical feature.

In most patients, diagnosis is made by nasal swabs obtained through the external nares. These usually reveal large numbers of capsulated yeast-like organisms, easily detected with most staining procedures. Although a non-species-specific latex cryptococcal antigen agglutination titre (LCAT) can be performed, generally it is regarded as an aid in the assessment of therapeutic efficacy, not so much as a diagnostic tool.

Aspergillosis and penicilliosis

Aspergillosis and penicilliosis are predominantly diseases of the dog. The majority of affected animals are younger than 7 years, and brachycephalic breeds are rarely affected. In most cases, the disease remains confined to the nasal cavity. Due to the fungi's tendency to cause vasculitis and secondary ischaemic necrosis, infection tends to result in turbinate destruction and loss of intranasal structures.

The most common clinical signs are chronic, profuse, sanguinopurulent nasal discharge with sneezing and epistaxis. The severity of the nasal discharge helps to differentiate this condition from nasal neoplasia, where the discharge tends to be less voluminous and often not quite as haemorrhagic or have had a longer period of prior non-haemorrhagic nasal discharge. Discomfort around the nostrils, mouth or bridge of the nose and face is commonly encountered as are ulcerations or excoriations of the external nares. These superficial abnormalities are uncommon in nasal neoplasia.

The diagnosis of aspergillosis or penicilliosis should be confirmed by at least two independent methods to avoid false positive or negative results. Diagnostic imaging is generally most rewarding. Loss of turbinate pattern and a general increase in radiolucency are seen with aspergillosis or penicilliosis due to turbinate necrosis. Nasal neoplasia may also produce turbinate destruction; however, the increased soft tissue and exudate generally produce an increase in radiodensity as well as a loss of the fine turbinate structures.

Rhinoscopy usually allows visualisation of fungal colonies. Rhinoscopy is particularly rewarding in cases of aspergillosis or penicilliosis, as turbinate and blood vessel destruction produces a large non-bleeding space. Fungal colonies are visualised as greenish-white plaques growing on turbinate mucosa and are easily biopsied for culture or cytological evaluation.

In the author's opinion, serology is generally unhelpful as both sensitivity and specificity are low (high numbers of false negatives and false positives, respectively). When they are used, they *must* always be interpreted in the light of the imaging and rhinoscopy results.

Non-infectious inflammatory causes

Non-infectious inflammatory causes of sneezing and nasal discharge are not uncommon in dogs and cats. Lymphocytic-plasmacytic rhinitis and allergic rhinitis are difficult to confirm, with the diagnosis usually made based on the demonstration of nasal mucosal biopsies revealing mononuclear cell infiltrates in patients with minimal structural changes and no evidence of mass lesions or other explanations for this sub-acute sterile inflammation.

Nasopharyngeal polyps

These are benign growths that have been mainly reported in kittens and young adult cats. The clinical signs are usually upper airway obstruction, noisy breathing and serous to mucopurulent nasal discharge.

Neoplasia

Various neoplastic disorders may cause a nasal discharge, including squamous cell carcinoma, fibrosarcoma, lymphoma and various adenocarcinomas. Most nasal tumours in dogs and cats are malignant, and prognosis is poor (except perhaps nasal lymphoma in cats).

Dyspnoea with minimal coughing

Define the location

Dyspnoeic animals with minimal coughing clearly have compromised respiratory function, and hence the answer to the question 'what system is involved?' must be – the respiratory system. The answer to the question 'what part of the respiratory system?' is a little more problematic but generally is going to fall into two fairly broad categories: those with dyspnoea and minimal coughing produced by laryngeal dysfunction and those with dyspnoea and minimal coughing produced by various intrathoracic disorders. Remember – only *rarely* do animals with predominantly tracheal disease present with dyspnoea as a major problem.

- Dyspnoea with minimal coughing suggests laryngeal or various forms of intrathoracic disease
- Patients with *laryngeal* dysfunction have predominantly *inspiratory* dyspnoea and *rarely cough* unless there is secondary tracheal irritation
- Patients with various forms of *intrathoracic* disease are more likely to have *expiratory* dyspnoea

Initial differentiation of these two broad regions of the respiratory tract is essential if the most effective diagnostic aids are to be used. This differentiation is best achieved, at least initially, through auscultation. By localising the area where the respiratory sounds are most audible, it is often possible to differentiate laryngeal from intrathoracic causes of dyspnoea. Furthermore, laryngeal dysfunction may produce a stridor (high pitched sound heard during inspiration) as well as dysphonia and occasionally deglutition problems.

Later in the course of disorders resulting in laryngeal dysfunction, severely affected cases may develop cyanosis and respiratory distress. The respiratory distress is a result of upper airway obstruction. Typically, it occurs during inspiration, as negative intra-airway pressures tend to suck surrounding tissues into the airway lumen. Expiration is often rapid and effortless.

Laryngeal disorders producing dyspnoea with minimal coughing

Cases with suspected primary laryngeal disease require thorough inspection of the caudal pharynx and larynx (laryngoscopy). Laryngoscopy allows visualisation of the larynx and pharynx for assessment of structural and functional abnormalities of the arytenoid cartilages and vocal cords. As functional problems need to be considered, restraint without pharmacological modification of laryngeal function is imperative.

Appropriate sedation

Generally, a light dose (2–4 mg/kg) of propofol given to effect is a reliable means of avoiding anaesthetic-induced 'excitement' and examining the area thoroughly in a suitably tractable patient. Both a laryngoscope and a small rigid endoscope help in illuminating the region and enhancing visualisation. The animal should be in sternal recumbency to minimise any asymmetry due to positioning.

Interestingly, one recent study has suggested that light thiopentone anaesthesia was preferable to propofol (with or without acepromazine), ketamine iv and diazepam iv, as all of these drugs affected arytenoid movement on inspiration. Because the study involved the use of a videoendoscope, thus necessitating a deeper plane of anaesthesia than required for direct visualisation of the larynx, it is possible that at lighter planes of anaesthesia, the agent effect would be less and of course the risk of anaesthetic-induced excitement when thiopentone is used, greater.

Once laryngeal function has been assessed, anaesthesia should be deepened and the caudal pharynx and larynx examined for structural abnormalities, foreign bodies or tumours and where appropriate samples obtained for histopathology.

Secondary changes

It should be remembered that prolonged upper airway obstruction results in the soft tissues being 'dragged' into the lumen by increased negative pressure. Eversion of the laryngeal saccules, thickening and elongation of the soft palate and inflammation with thickening of the pharyngeal and laryngeal mucosa can occur. The laryngeal cartilages can become soft and deformed and in severe cases collapse medially resulting in variably occluded air flow.

4 Define the lesion

Laryngeal disorders commonly encountered in companion animal practice can be broadly classified under the following pathological processes:

- inflammatory
- malformations
- degenerative
- neoplastic
- paresis.

Intrathoracic disorders producing dyspnoea with minimal coughing

When dyspnoea is present with minimal or absent coughing and laryngeal function appears and auscultates normally, various intrathoracic disorders should be considered. Specifically, these are likely to be the following:

- space-occupying disorders of the pleural cavity
- constrictive bronchial inflammation
- various cardiac disorders.

In animals with intrathoracic disorders, auscultation can be particularly helpful in a logical approach to investigation of the problem. In order to more fully appreciate the benefits of thorough thoracic auscultation, it is worth remembering how and where auscultatable thoracic respiratory sounds are generated.

Normal lung sounds

Normally, thoracic auscultation reveals bronchial and vesicular sounds. Bronchial sounds are tubular sounds similar to those heard over the trachea and are more prominent in the hilar areas. Vesicular sounds are likened to 'wind through the trees', are softer and are heard more peripherally.

Abnormal lung sounds

Abnormal lung sounds can be amplified tubular or vesicular sounds, 'crackles' or 'wheezes'.

- Crackles are non-musical, discontinuous noises similar to cellophane being crumpled or bubbles popping. Crackles are usually associated with relatively viscous fluid within airways.
- Wheezes are more musical, continuous high-pitched whistling sounds. Wheezes suggest narrowing of airway diameters through the presence of excessive amounts of material such as exudate, thickening of the airway walls, active bronchoconstriction or increased compliance of the airways resulting in their collapse whenever there is a significant increase in intrathoracic pressure (e.g. with expiration).

As can be seen from the above-mentioned descriptions, abnormal thoracic respiratory sounds are predominantly produced by turbulent air movement in the *airways*. In an animal with dyspnoea and minimal coughing that has relatively normal laryngeal auscultation, thoracic auscultation is likely to be very helpful in differentiating the three broad categories of intrathoracic disorder likely to be causing the problem.

Space-occupying disorders of the pleural cavity

Space-occupying disorders of the pleural cavity may include the presence of significant amounts of air, fluid, ectopic normal organs or abnormal tissues. The clinician may be alerted to the presence of a space-occupying lesion in the pleural space by a dulling or muffling of respiratory sounds. The contrast is highlighted in a dyspnoeic animal where increased respiratory sounds would be expected due to increased volume and velocity of air flowing through airways.

In situations where there are clinically significant amounts of material in the pleural space, although there is increased movement of the chest wall, the lungs are not expanding normally, reducing the volume and velocity of air flow. This and the greater distance between the lungs (and more specifically the 'sound-generating bronchii') and the chest wall, combine to produce muffled respiratory sounds on thoracic auscultation.

Diagnostic procedures

Patients with suspected pleural effusions require *radiology or CT scan* and *ultrasonography* of the thorax to document the magnitude of the effusion and to define any potential solid tissue masses in the pleural space. The detection of solid tissue within the pleural cavity should be further evaluated by *fine needle aspirates* whenever possible.

Thoracocentesis is another valuable aid in determining the nature and possible aetiology of the pleural fluid. However, it should always be remembered that any pleural effusion is likely to produce bizarre reactive mesothelial cells, which may be mistaken for poorly differentiated neoplastic cells.

Should I remove the fluid?

In some severely affected individuals, removal of pleural fluid may be critical, and this should be considered once thoracic ultrasonography has been performed. Fluid removal may also provide improved radiological definition of the pleural structures. Significant amounts of pleural fluid are most conveniently and thoroughly removed using surgically implanted chest drains.

4 Define the lesion

Space-occupying lesion of the pleural cavity will be composed of various fluids (including blood, chyle, transudates and exudates) as well as transposed normal tissues and abnormal tissues such as neoplasms. Pleural fluid characterisation can be clarifying in determining possible causes.

- Inflammatory exudate suggests a primary inflammatory process.
- Transudates suggest increased systemic venous pressure or decreased oncotic pressure, although the latter is usually associated with generalised oedema.
- Chylous effusions can also develop as a result of increased systemic venous pressure or due to disturbances in the thoracic lymphatic drainage for any reason at all.
    - In dogs as with most other animals, when the venous hypertension is caused by heart failure, this will be due to increased *right* atrial pressure and thus right heart failure.
    - In cats, when the thoracic venous hypertension is caused by heart failure transudates and chylous effusions, this may be due to increased *left* atrial pressure.
- Haemorrhagic thoracic effusions are usually a sign of neoplasia or recent trauma.

While cytology and fluid analysis can be helpful in determining possible causes for thoracic effusions, ultrasonography is likely to be the most rewarding diagnostic aid in clarifying potentially displaced normal or simply abnormal structures present in the thoracic cavity. This is particularly true if there is some pleural effusion to increase the acoustic window.

Constrictive bronchial inflammation

4 Define the lesion

While many bronchial disorders will result in varying degrees of coughing, few are likely to result in dyspnoea with minimal coughing.

The one notable exception to this generalisation is those disorders of the smaller bronchii characterised by marked bronchospasm. Because the overall diameter of the bronchial system will be reduced, these animals will have dyspnoea as a marked clinical characteristic, and if the cause for the bronchospasm does not illicit an exudative response, there will be minimal coughing. Due to the turbulence in airflow created by the luminal narrowing, patients will have dramatically increased airway sounds and hence increased thoracic respiratory sounds, which are frequently generalised.

By far, the most common type of pathology resulting in generalised narrowing of the diameter of the bronchial tree is the constrictive inflammation seen as a result of the release of various inflammatory cytokines, which stimulate bronchoconstriction. Interestingly, this is almost exclusively seen in cats and not dogs, as the latter generally do not release 'bronchonconstricting cytokines' in response to airway inflammation. Hence, most dogs with bronchial inflammation will not be characterised by bronchoconstriction and thus do not present with dyspnoea and minimal coughing.

Diagnostic procedures

Diagnostic procedures that may be helpful include the following:

- Thoracic imaging: this might include thoracic radiology or CT. However, as dyspnoea with minimal coughing due to bronchial disease is likely to be predominantly constrictive inflammation with minimal exudates present, the chest is likely to appear normal regardless of the imaging modality. Indeed, with standard thoracic radiography, the airways may be difficult to find due to general pulmonary over-inflation. However, the presence of a normal thoracic radiograph in a cat with marked dyspnoea and minimal coughing with normal laryngeal and cardiac auscultation and generalised, increased thoracic respiratory sounds is strongly suggestive of constrictive bronchial inflammation.
- Transtracheal aspirate
- Bronchial wash/bronchoalveolar lavage
- Haematology.

Various cardiac disorders

When dyspnoea with minimal coughing is due to compromised cardiac function, cardiac abnormalities are also likely to be detectable.

These may include the following:

- Alterations in palpable or audible cardiac impulse
- Reduced pulse amplitude
- Tachyarrhythmias
- Murmurs consistent with mitral insufficiency, aortic stenosis or murmurs suggesting left to right shunting.

These manifestations of cardiac dysfunction can be supported by echocardiographic evidence for alterations in normal cardiac structures as well as estimation of circulating levels of various neuropeptides, which are likely to be elevated in animals with respiratory dysfunction secondary to heart failure and not elevated in animals with respiratory dysfunction that is *not* secondary to heart failure.

Coughing

Define the system

The act of coughing is a forced expiratory effort against an initially closed glottis, which then opens, resulting in the explosive release of air from the lungs through the larynx and mouth. There is generally an initial increased inspiration before the cough, allowing the respiratory muscles to work to greater mechanical advantage. The pressure that builds up behind the closed glottis can reach 40 kPa and, if often repeated, can lead to significant reductions in venous return with syncope being an unusual but dramatic consequence.

The cough reflex is initiated by irritant and mechanical receptors predominantly located in the trachea and major bronchi. The receptors can be activated by irritation from mucus, dust, foreign material or chemical irritation, as well as sudden or marked changes in airway lumen diameter.

Clearly, in a patient with coughing, the answer to the question 'what system is involved?' must be – *the respiratory system*. This is important to remember, especially in small animal practice where the presence of myxomatous mitral valve degeneration (MMVD) is a common problem in mature dogs. As stated previously, there is always a tendency to attribute a particular problem to a single disorder. Hence, the detection of MMVD in a coughing dog makes the assumption that the coughing is due to cardiac disease appealing. However, many dogs with MMVD have no clinical signs for long periods after the valve dysfunction is detected through an audible murmur. In other words, while explaining two abnormal findings with one disease is attractive, in this case, it will not always be appropriate, and it is essential that all aspects of the history and physical examination be used to make this assessment.

Perhaps, a more logical way of approaching the problem is as follows. Coughing is a sign of respiratory disease. One cause of this respiratory disease might be pulmonary congestion due to left-sided heart failure brought about by MMVD. However, for MMVD to cause heart failure and thus coughing due to pulmonary congestion and oedema, there needs to be some level of *heart failure* and hence recruitment of the principal compensatory mechanisms – activation of the sympathetic nervous system and the rennin-angiotensin system. The former of course, being more easily recognisable on physical examination. Thus, the absence of any evidence to suggest recruitment of such compensatory processes (e.g. a lack of tachycardia or the presence of a sinus arrhythmia) should alert the clinician to the likelihood that the coughing is *not* a consequence of the MMVD.

While coughing is clearly a sign of respiratory system involvement, the next step in a logical approach to its investigation – answering the question 'what part of the respiratory system is involved?' can be substantially facilitated by dividing coughing patients into those associated with dyspnoea and those where dyspnoea is minimal or inconsequential.

Coughing with minimal dyspnoea

3 Define the location

Coughing with minimal dyspnoea is generally associated with *tracheal or large airway* disease. Disorders of these structures often produce coughing that has a harsh 'hacking' sound, will frequently occur in paroxysms and may be followed by retching. Whenever bronchial disease is present, thoracic auscultation invariably results in audible wheezes and crackles being detected on thoracic auscultation, with more severely affected areas usually indicated by more prominent sounds from the affected area(s).

Many of the disorders that affect the trachea and large airways will not be associated with dyspnoea, as it is difficult to significantly occlude the lumen of these relatively wide airways. Although uncommon, there is however *one* exception, *tracheal hypoplasia*. This is a congenital malformation of the trachea that results in a significant narrowing of the trachea generally starting at the thoracic inlet and affecting varying amounts of the cranial part of the intrathoracic trachea. The reduction in luminal diameter can be dramatic, and in many cases, this can result in varying degrees of dyspnoea. This is an uncommon disorder and has been reported to be over-represented in a number of brachycephalic breeds and Rhodesian ridgebacks.

When the bronchial tree is involved in cases of coughing with minimal dyspnoea, there is likely to be minimal narrowing of the *overall* diameter of the bronchial system. In addition, while disorders that affect the bronchi may be associated with coughing and minimal dyspnoea, certain bronchial disorders may be more likely to produce coughing *and* dyspnoea or, as indicated previously, dyspnoea with minimal coughing. In cats, in particular, inflammation of the airways due to various hypersensitivities produces inflammation and varying degrees of bronchospasm characterised by dyspnoea, which is usually expiratory.

In other words, depending on the type of lesion or pathology, bronchial disease may present with predominantly coughing, predominantly dyspnoea or both.

4 Define the lesion

As previously mentioned, disorders of the trachea and large bronchi usually result in coughing with minimal dyspnoea. In addition, disorders of these structures often produce coughing that has a harsh 'hacking' sound, will frequently occur in paroxysms and may be followed by retching.

Coughing with minimal dyspnoea suggests tracheal involvement and possibly bronchial disorders with no or minimal luminal narrowing.

The most common types of pathology affecting the trachea and bronchi that are likely to result in coughing and minimal dyspnoea include the following:

- Malformations: including disorders such as bronchiectasis and ciliary dyskinesis
- Exudative inflammation
  - inflammation likely to result in varying degrees of exudate, which will stimulate airway-located cough receptors.
- Degenerative disorders of the cartilage supporting the trachea and bronchii resulting in chondromalacia (collapsing trachea, collapsing bronchii) and increased likelihood of irritation through contact of adjacent areas of luminal mucosa because of the inability of these airways to maintain patency. Despite variously held perceptions, this inability *tends to result in coughing with minimal dyspnoea.*
- Neoplasia
  - disruption of airflow and potential erosion of the regional mucoasa are all likely to stimulate the relevant cough receptors. Although bronchial neoplasia may occlude the affected bronchi, the overall diameter of the bronchial system is unlikely to be compromised until later in the course of the disease, and hence animals are likely to first present with coughing and minimal dyspnoea.

Diagnostic procedures

Patients with coughing and minimal dyspnoea are likely to have tracheobronchial disease and usually require various diagnostic steps to be performed to evaluate and characterise their dysfunction. The notable exception to this statement is the common and generally self-limiting canine tracheobronchial disorder, infectious tracheopbronchitis, where the history and physical findings are particularly characteristic, and its self-limiting nature generally justifies a 'wait and see with perhaps some supportive therapy' approach.

Diagnostic procedures that may be helpful include the following:

- Thoracic imaging.
  - This might include thoracic radiology or CT.

- Although the more common disorders affecting the trachea are rarely visualised using standard imaging, there may be indications of increased smaller airway radiodensity (bronchial pattern); however, this may not always be apparent. In fact, as coughing with minimal dyspnoea may occur as a result of functional changes in the large airways, dynamic evaluation of the airways will be essential in certain situations, and hence ideally fluoroscopy (cine-radiography) should always be a potential part of any diagnostic evaluation.

- Tracheoscopy/bronchoscopy
  - especially if cine-radiography is not available
- Cytology from affected airways
  - as many of these diseases will require cytology from either trans-tracheal aspirate, bronchial wash or bronchoalveolar lavage.

Coughing accompanied by dyspnoea

Define the location

Coughing accompanied by dyspnoea is most often a reflection of pulmonary parenchymal disease or, as described previously, certain forms of bronchial disease. In contrast to laryngeal disease, where the dyspnoea tends to be more inspiratory, the dyspnoea associated with bronchopulmonary disease tends to be most notable on expiration or throughout inspiration and expiration.

The forms of bronchopulmonary problems likely to produce coughing and dyspnoea may also result in the increased presence of excessive amounts of fluid within the respiratory system. The presence of this increased fluid can mean the coughing tends to be productive.

Productive coughing sounds 'moist' and results in mucus, exudate, oedema fluid or blood from airways being delivered to the oral cavity. Usually, the animals demonstrably swallow the material. Rarely, expectoration occurs and can be confused with vomiting. In addition, the resultant modification of airway diameter that can occur as a result of this material being present along with the increased respiratory effort is likely to result in increased thoracic respiratory sounds as discussed previously.

> Almost all animals with bronchial or pulmonary parenchymal disease resulting in coughing and dyspnoea will have abnormalities on careful and thorough thoracic auscultation.

Patients with coughing accompanied by dyspnoea usually require some combination of the following diagnostic procedures for further elucidation of their bronchopulmonary disease:

- Thoracic imaging with either radiography or preferably CT
- Bronchial washings
- Transtracheal washings
- Transthoracic pulmonary aspirates
- 'Systemic' tests for pulmonary parasitic diseases
- Arterial blood gas analysis
- Sampling for various infectious agents such as *Dirofilaria immitus* serology or faecal examination for *Angiostrongylus* larvae
- When there is a consideration as to whether the disorder is due to heart failure, sampling for estimating N-terminal pro-B-type natriuretic peptide (NT-pro-BNP)
- Thoracoscopy and/or open-chest lung biopsy.

The choice of the above-mentioned diagnostic aids will depend on the likely aetiology or aetiologies and typical pathological processes engendered.

Define the lesion

The types of pathological processes likely to affect the pulmonary parenchyma include the following:

- Inflammation: which might be infectious or non-infectious
- Thromboembolism: which might be due to primary pulmonary arterial disease such as occurs with dirofilariasis or might be secondary to systemic disorders resulting in hypercoaguable states such as diffuse inflammatory processes or disorders resulting in reduced levels of thrombolytic products such as protein-losing nephropathies
- Pulmonary congestion and oedema: by far, the most common reason for this being left-sided heart failure

- Neoplasia
- Degenerative fibrosis, which currently remains an idiopathic process
- Emphysema: generally a result of chronic collapsing airway disease or severe degenerative pathology.

Inflammatory pulmonary parenchymal disease

Inflammatory pulmonary parenchymal disease can be classified as *infectious* or *non-infectious (immune mediated)*. The cause of the parenchymal inflammation should be established, as therapy for the various immune-mediated inflammatory problems will be contraindicated in those cases with an infectious aetiology.

Infectious causes

The various causes of *infectious* pulmonary parenchymal disease include the following:

- Viral
  - Several viruses can infect the lower respiratory tract, but viral pneumonia rarely dominates the clinical picture.
  - Occasionally, feline corona virus infection may present with predominantly pulmonary signs, although thorough investigation usually reveals evidence for multi-system disease. Feline calicivirus and herpesvirus have rarely been associated with pulmonary inflammation.
- Bacterial
  - A variety of bacteria can infect the lung.
  - Generally, gram-negative facultative anaerobic bacilli and intestinal anaerobes predominate.
  - It is worth noting that bacterial pneumonia is usually associated with an underlying process causing altered pharyngeo-oesophageal function or persistent vomiting, immuno-incompetence or functional/structural abnormalities within the respiratory tract such as bronchiectasis, ciliary dyskinesia, thromboembolic disease, neoplasia or, of course, foreign bodies.
  - Common isolates include *Pasteurella, Klebsiella, Escherichia, Pseudomonas, Staphylococci* and *Streptococci*.

- Fungal
  - Mycotic causes of pneumonia are not particularly common except in certain parts of North America and rarely produce signs consistent with pulmonary parenchymal disease *alone*.
  - Most cases present with evidence for multi-system disease.
  - Occasionally, individuals with immuno-incompetence may be susceptible to a number of different organisms with relatively low virulence such as cryptococcosis or pneumocystis.
- Parasitic
  - In many parts of the world, the most common cause of parasitic pulmonary inflammation is dirofilariasis, a common cause of eosinophilic pneumonitis.
  - Infectious dirofilariasis probably produces eosinophilic pneumonitis by antibody-dependent leucocyte adherence to microfilaria, which are subsequently trapped in the pulmonary capillaries and removed through the pulmonary reticuloendothelial system. This tends to produce granulomatous inflammation, which may resemble sterile, immune-mediated eosinophilic pneumonitis or may progress to massive pulmonary granulomas, usually with marked hilar lymphadenomegaly.
  - Other parasites that may cause pulmonary disease include *Aelurostrongylus abstrusus* (cats) and *Angiostrongylus vasorum*.
  - In the United Kingdom and Europe, perhaps the most common cause of parasitic pneumonia is that caused by *Angiostrongylus vasorum*. This parasitic infestation can produce various degrees of pulmonary inflammation, as well as unexplained but clinically significant coagulopathies.

Diagnostic procedures

Diagnostic procedures that may be helpful include the following:

- Thoracic imaging
  - This might include thoracic radiology or CT.
  - Most infectious inflammatory conditions will result in either exudative or granulomatous inflammation resulting in either an alveolar or nodular pattern of increased radio-density of the pulmonary parenchyma, respectively.
  - The type of pattern and its distribution can certainly provide clues as to the underlying reasons for the problem. For instance,

because of the early opening of the right apical lobar bronchus, aspiration of oral/gastric contents frequently affect the right apical lobe.
    - Aspirated foreign bodies are likely to produce rather severe but relatively well-defined regions of increased radio-density with a well-defined alveolar pattern.
- Cytology and culture via transtracheal aspirate or bronchial washings
    - In many cases, transtracheal aspirate provides a definitive diagnosis without the need for an anaesthetic.
    - Obtaining a sample for culture should generally be attempted before starting antimicrobial therapy.
- Haematology
    - A peripheral leukogram may reflect the inflammatory process, although a normal leukogram does not preclude septic pneumonia.

Non-infectious pulmonary parenchymal inflammation

Non-infectious inflammatory bronchopulmonary disorders are generally a manifestation of a primary disorder of the animal's immune system with an ill-defined underlying cause. In general terms, these tend to manifest themselves as exudative or granulomatous bronchopulmonary inflammation with the former being far more common.

The exudative disorders tend to result in sterile pulmonary infiltrates often, but not always, rich in eosinophils. They probably represent a variety of hypersensitivity disorders of the lung. The inciting agent is often difficult to establish, although pulmonary parasitism is frequently incriminated. Dogs and cats of all ages are affected, and usually systemic signs are mild or absent.

The granulomatous disorders result in multiple nodular inflammation, which destroys the underlying pulmonary architecture. The term 'lymphomatoid granulomatosis' has been used to describe this form of immune-mediated bronchopulmonary inflammation.

Diagnostic procedures

Diagnostic procedures that may be helpful include the following:

- Thoracic imaging
    - This might include thoracic radiology or CT.

  - As the radiographic appearance can be identical to the inflammatory changes seen with infectious causes, imaging rarely helps in determining whether the inflammation is a primary immune-mediated problem or a result of an infectious agent.
  - Depending on the type of immune-mediated process, there will usually be an increased radiodensity of the pulmonary parenchyma with an interstitial or mixed alveolar and interstitial pattern.
  - Granulomatous immune-mediated bronchopulmonary disease is characterised by large nodular densities visible throughout the pulmonary parenchyma.
  - Hilar lymphadenomegaly is often present in the more severely affected animals.
- Cytology and culture via transtracheal aspirate or bronchial washings:
  - On occasions, the cytology will be strongly suggestive of a non-infectious aetiology, especially if there are large numbers of eosinophils present while the granulomatous forms produce large numbers of lymphocytes and plasma cells without significant numbers of eosinophils.
  - Consequently, it is difficult to differentiate lymphomatoid granulomatosis from pulmonary neoplasia, mycotic pneumonitis or even atypical bacterial pneumonitis. Diagnosis must be made through tissue biopsy of the nodules, which may require fluoroscopically guided needle biopsies or samples obtained through thoracoscopy or even thoracotomy.
  - Of course, the material obtained will be sterile and with no evidence of intracellular bacteria or the presence of parasites either in the washings or on the basis of serology or faecal examination.

Thromboembolic pulmonary parenchymal disease

Thromboemboli generally form as a result of disease in organs other than the lungs. Circulating emboli such as bacteria, fat, air, parasites and circulating parts of thrombi from elsewhere in the body can be trapped in the pulmonary vascular system.

Thrombi can develop within vessels as a result of the following:

- venous stasis
- turbulent blood flow
- endothelial damage
- systemic hypercoagulability.

Thrombi are usually eliminated soon after formation, although this balance may become disturbed in many disease states. The most common conditions associated with thromboembolism include the following:

- dirofilariasis
- hyperlipidaemia
- hyperadrenocorticism
- hypothyroidism
- glomerulopathies
- immune-mediated haemolytic anaemia
- pancreatitis
- DIC.

The interference in pulmonary blood flow caused by the thromboemboli results in *ventilation-perfusion abnormalities* producing hypoxaemia and hypo-, normo- or hypercapnia, depending on the degree of respiratory drive. As carbon dioxide is far more soluble than oxygen, the absence of hypocapnia in an hypoxic patient suggests severe compromised respiratory function and generally a grave prognosis. Pulmonary hypertension may occur acutely with massive obstruction or reflex vasoconstriction. This occurs more commonly in chronic cases with recurrent disease. Pulmonary infarction is relatively uncommon.

The sudden onset of hypoxia produces peracute dyspnoea and tachypnoea, which will tend to be followed by coughing within 1–5 days. In cases with recurrent disease, there may be right cardiomegaly or split second heart sounds – evidence for pulmonary hypertension.

Diagnostic procedures

Diagnostic procedures that may be helpful include the following:

- Thoracic imaging
  - This might include radiography and/or CT imaging.
  - Unless the disorder has a chronic history, thoracic radiographs are normal, despite severe respiratory signs and blood gas evidence for marked ventilation-perfusion abnormalities.
  - Such inconsistency is highly suspicious for pulmonary vascular disease.
  - In more sub-acute or chronic cases, truncated pulmonary arteries occasionally ending in focal areas of interstitial or alveolar radiodensities are rare pathognomonic signs.

- More commonly, definitive diagnosis requires angiographic demonstration of truncation and/or intravascular filling defects.
  - The sensitivity of this technique is substantially enhanced if CT angiography can be used.

Pulmonary oedema

In most animals, pulmonary oedema is usually a result of clinically significant *left-sided heart failure* resulting in left atrial hypertension, pulmonary venous hypertension, pulmonary congestion and ultimately pulmonary oedema. Any cardiac disease that results in left atrial hypertension may produce pulmonary oedema. By far, the most common causes in small animal practice are the acquired cardiac disorders myxomatous degenerative mitral valve disease and dilated cardiomyopathy in dogs and hypertrophic cardiomyopathy in the cat.

Less commonly, increased pulmonary vascular permeability or reduced plasma oncotic pressure may be the underlying explanation. When reduced plasma oncotic pressure is the inciting agent, pulmonary oedema is likely to be just one manifestation of generalised subcutaneous oedema.

In addition, pulmonary oedema may occur with high output cardiac disease with no left atrial hypertension. The marked increase in pulmonary blood flow results in extravasation of fluid at a rate that exceeds pulmonary lymphatic capacitance. This form of high output pulmonary oedema may occur in some congenital cardiac anomalies such as patent ductus arteriosis or ventricular septal defect.

Neurogenic pulmonary oedema results from massive sympathetic stimulation. The sympathetic discharge raises peripheral resistance and systemic blood pressure resulting in a massive shift in blood volume from the systemic to pulmonary circulation. Pulmonary venous pressure rises dramatically and fluid is extravasated. Both central venous and pulmonary venous pressures usually return to normal within 30 minutes avoiding acute heart failure. However, the hypertension and hypervolaemia damage the capillary endothelium causing increased permeability and persistence of pulmonary oedema.

In *adult respiratory distress syndrome*, pulmonary oedema occurs due to increased pulmonary capillary permeability without an increase in pulmonary venous pressure. It is a common response of the lung to many forms of injury. The abnormalities in permeability that occur are the result of damage to alveolar epithelial and microvascular barriers. Multiple mediators are likely to be involved in causing increased permeability and include endotoxins (directly toxic to vascular endothelium), various inflammatory mediators (cytokines and eicosanoids) as well as excessive levels of platelets and platelet-activating factor. These mechanisms can be activated by many conditions, including inhaled toxins, sepsis, pancreatitis, aspirating gastric contents and various drugs.

Whatever the cause of the pulmonary oedema, fluid initially accumulates in the interstitium, then rapidly spreads to alveolar spaces and in severe cases, the airways. Respiratory function is adversely affected as alveolar compression and reduced surfactant create atelectasis and decreased pulmonary compliance. Furthermore, regional hypoxia and hypocapnia produce constriction of pulmonary arterioles and bronchioles, respectively. These constrictive processes are exacerbated by a general increase in interstitial pressure.

Diagnostic procedures

Diagnostic procedures that may be helpful include the following:

- Thoracic imaging
  - There is increased pulmonary parenchymal radiodensity with an alveolar pattern and a perivascular distribution.
  - In dogs, pulmonary oedema due to left heart failure and thus left atrial hypertension is frequently more pronounced in the perihilar regions of the caudal lung lobes. Interestingly, this does not appear to be the case in cats where the alveolar radiodensity's distribution is far less predictable.
- When the pulmonary oedema is due to left atrial hypertension, cardiac abnormalities are also likely to be detectable and may include the following:
  - Alterations in palpable or audible cardiac impulse
  - Reduced pulse amplitude
  - Tachyarrhythmias
  - Murmurs consistent with mitral insufficiency, aortic stenosis or murmurs suggesting left to right shunting.

These manifestations of cardiac dysfunction can be supported by radiographic or echocardiographic evidence for alterations in normal cardiac structures as well as estimation of circulating levels of various neuropeptides, which are likely to be elevated in animals with respiratory dysfunction secondary to heart failure and not elevated in animals with respiratory dysfunction that is *not* secondary to heart failure. All of this information, of course, *must* be interpreted in the light of the presence or absence of significant non-cardiac intrathoracic disease.

Pulmonary neoplasia

Primary pulmonary tumours, metastatic neoplasia and multi-centric neoplasia can all involve the pulmonary parenchyma.

Although most primary pulmonary tumours are malignant, metastases are not common in the early phases of the disease; consequently, complete surgical removal provides an opportunity for a significant post-operative period of remission. Unfortunately, clinical signs may not be obvious until there has been significant involvement of the pulmonary parenchyma, as the onset of coughing and dyspnoea is usually chronic and slowly progressive. However, on occasions, peracute manifestations may occur with complications such as pneumothorax or thromboembolism.

Diagnostic procedures

Diagnostic procedures that may be helpful include the following:

- Thoracic imaging
  - Thoracic radiography or CT frequently reveals focal areas of increased radiodensity with obliteration of all underlying structures.
  - Margins are often distinct, and cavitation may be present.
  - Metastatic or multi-centric disease results in a diffuse interstitial pattern with or without nodular changes.
- Cytology
  - a tissue diagnosis may be achieved by bronchial washings or bronchoalveolar lavage, although direct tissue biopsy is often required.

Degenerative fibrosis

This is a poorly understood condition, which is assumed to be a low-grade immune-mediated inflammatory disorder, which results in progressive fibrosis of the pulmonary parenchyma. It is almost exclusively encountered in dogs and is markedly over-represented in small white breeds such as West Highland white terriers and Maltese.

This condition could be considered as an intrathoracic cause for dyspnoea with minimal coughing, as this may indeed be the way affected animals present early in the course of the disease. However, by the time most patients are afflicted the degenerative process has progressed and is more likely to result in dyspnoea with variable amounts of coughing, especially as affected animals are prone to developing secondary bronchopulmonary bacterial infections. Most affected individuals have generalised increased thoracic respiratory sounds with prominent crackles and wheezing.

Diagnostic procedures

Diagnostic procedures that may be helpful include the following:

- Thoracic imaging
  - Thoracic radiography or CT will generally be characterised by a diffuse increased radiodensity of the pulmonary parenchyma typical of a diffuse interstitial pattern.
- Tissue biopsies via thoracoscopy
  - Cytology is invariably non-diagnostic in these cases, so bronchial washings or bronchoalveolar lavage is generally unhelpful, and direct tissue biopsy is almost always required for a definitive diagnosis.

Emphysema

Emphysema specifically refers to the pathological process where there is rupture and coalescing of alveoli creating air saccules of larger volume. The resultant reduction in the surface area to volume ratio of these larger volume saccules results in impaired gas exchange, and once the changes become sufficiently significant, affected animals will develop increasing dyspnoea. While the emphysema itself is not likely to stimulate coughing, in small animals, this is an end-stage process as a result of chronic collapsing airway disease or severe degenerative pathology with associated bronchial disturbances resulting in both coughing and dyspnoea.

> All primary respiratory problems may produce some degree of pulmonary hypertension, which can result in secondary right cardiomegaly

Haemoptysis

Haemoptysis refers to expectoration of bloody material. While rarely this can be a sign of a systemic coagulopathy (see Chapter 11), in the majority of cases, it indicates primary structural respiratory disease. While any part of the respiratory tract distal to the larynx may result in haemoptysis, generally haemoptysis is indicative of significant structural bronchopulmonary disease and is most commonly associated with severe inflammatory disease secondary to bronchopulmonary neoplasia or severe parasitic infestations such as dirofilariasis or angiostrongylosis.

Cyanosis

Cyanosis is produced by an *absolute* increase in the quantity of unoxygenated haemoglobin. It generally reflects severe hypoxia, although because it is the level of unoxygenated haemoglobin rather than the percentage of haemoglobin unoxygenated, cyanosis can be present in an animal with marked polycythaemia and relatively normal oxygenation. While polycythemia can be an adaptive response to cardiorespiratory dysfunction resulting in impaired oxygen exchange, it may also be a result of primary haematopoietic disease. Thus cyanosis may be a result of primary or secondary respiratory dysfunction or primary haematopoietic dysfunction.

Classically, cyanosis has been thought of as reflecting significant right to left shunting of blood producing large amounts of unoxygenated haemoglobin in the systemic circulation. Consequently, in an animal with no other clinical signs, cyanosis is likely to be an indicator of a combination of ventricular or atrial septal defects with concurrent pulmonary hypertension. Characteristically, patent ductus arteriosus with pulmonary hypertension will tend to result in caudal and not cranial cyanosis. Another potent cause of cyanosis is laryngeal paralysis, and when this is bilateral, the degree of stridor may well be less obvious than might be imagined.

Conclusion

Clinical manifestations of respiratory system dysfunction are relatively limited, but there are a multitude of causes. Recognition of the importance of defining and refining the problem/location and appreciating that the respiratory system may be involved primarily or secondarily is crucial in the pathway to formulating a rational list of possible diagnoses and progressing understanding of the disorder by choosing appropriate diagnostic aids.

CHAPTER 9

Anaemia

Jill E. Maddison
The Royal Veterinary College, Department of Clinical Science and Services, London, UK

Anaemia is a relatively common clinical problem with a multitude of causes. It is characterised by a significant decrease of red blood cells (RBCs) and/or haemoglobin blood levels or oxygen–haemoglobin binding capacities. Its clinical importance can vary from being the patient's primary life-threatening problem to being relatively clinically inconsequential.

Define the problem

Animals with anaemia present with pale mucous membranes. The first step is, therefore, to define the problem and system involved – that is to differentiate those animals with pale mucous membranes due to poor peripheral perfusion (e.g. due to hypovolaemia, cardiogenic shock and pain) from those that have a reduced RBC mass. Animals with pale mucous membranes due to poor peripheral perfusion will often (but not always) have prolonged capillary refill times and/or weak femoral pulses.

Once it has been confirmed that 'true' anaemia is the cause of the animal's pale mucous membranes, it is important to assess whether the anaemia is the primary disease process or secondary, that is, is it causing the animal's presenting clinical signs or is it secondary to an underlying disorder. Often, the clinical significance of mild to moderate anaemia is overestimated. The most common cause of mild anaemia is anaemia of chronic disease, which is a feature of many infectious, inflammatory or neoplastic disorders (discussed later in the chapter).

Clinical Reasoning in Small Animal Practice, First Edition.
Jill E. Maddison, Holger A. Volk and David B. Church.

The assessment of clinical disease onset and progression is important to help differentiate possible causes. The rapidity with which anaemia develops will also influence its clinical effect. For example, a dog with a packed cell volume (PCV) of 20% may show only mild clinical signs if the anaemia has developed slowly but will be more severely affected if the PCV has decreased suddenly.

Assessment of anaemia

Unless the anaemia is clearly of acute onset, it is imperative to ascertain whether the anaemia is regenerative or non-regenerative. The diagnostic approach and possible aetiologies for regenerative and non-regenerative anaemia are by and large different (although there is some overlap), and full evaluation of the haemogram for clues relating to regeneration is essential.

Be aware, however, that it takes 2–4 days for the bone marrow to fully respond to acute anaemia, and therefore, signs of complete regeneration may not be present if peracute RBC loss (from haemorrhage or haemolysis) has occurred. However, usually within 24 hours, there will be some evidence of a response even if it is not complete.

The assessment of anaemia requires consideration of RBC parameters such as size as well as morphology. Evidence for regeneration includes the following:

- Increased RBC size – macrocytosis (increased mean corpuscular volume – MCV)
- Variation in RBC staining and size (polychromasia and anisocytosis; Figure 9.1)
- Presence of increased numbers of reticulocytes (Figure 9.2)
- Presence of nucleated RBC (although these can also occur with lead toxicity and splenic pathology; Figure 9.1)

RBC morphological abnormalities may assist in the assessment of possible causes. Cell changes of importance include the following:

- Spherocytosis (Figure 9.1)
  - Common in immune-mediated haemolytic anaemia (IMHA), but small numbers can be hereditary (rare) or occur in patients with a mononuclear phagocytic neoplasm, microangiopathic haemolysis, zinc toxicity and hypophosphataemia

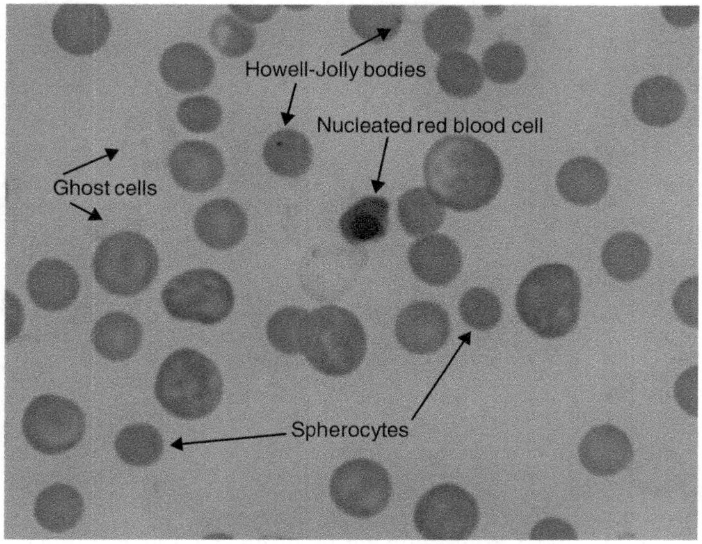

Figure 9.1 A blood smear from a dog with immune mediated haemolytic anaemia with strong evidence of regeneration, including anisocytosis and polychromasia (variations in size and staining of red bloods cells), nucleated red blood cells, Howell-Jolly bodies. The smear also shows numerous spherocytes and ghost cells (indicating extravascular and intravascular haemolysis, respectively). Wright's stain. *Reproduced with permission of Dr Balazs Szladovits.*

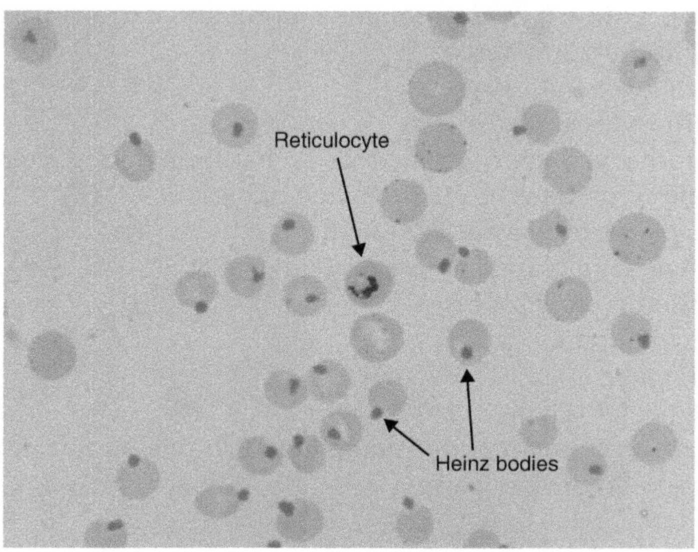

Figure 9.2 Blood smear from a cat with reticulocytes and numerous Heinz bodies. New Methylene Blue stain. *Reproduced with permission of Dr Balazs Szladovits.*

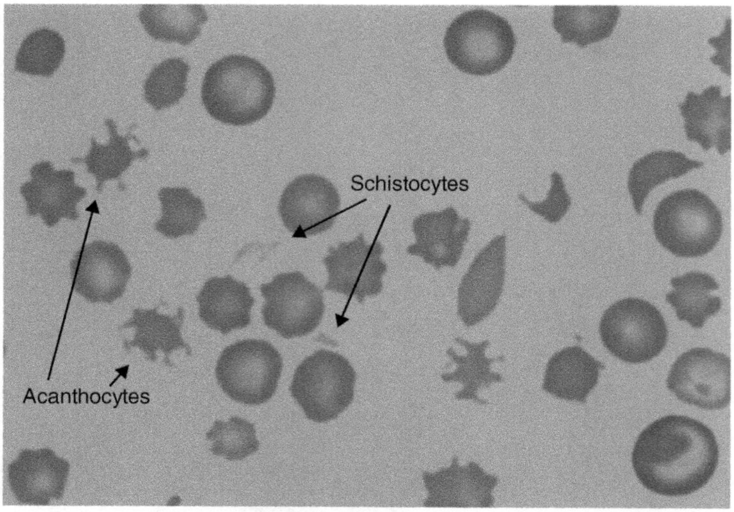

Figure 9.3 Blood smear from a dog with schistocytes and acanthocytes indicating shear damage to the erythrocytes. Wright's stain. *Reproduced with permission of Dr Balazs Szladovits.*

- Shistocytosis (Figure 9.3)
  - Shistocytes are RBC fragments that have resulted from blood being either forced through abnormally narrow passages or physically traumatised.
  - See Table 9.1 for causes
- Acanthocytosis (Figure 9.3)
  - Acanthocytes are spiculated RBCs that form due to altered lipid: cholesterol ratios in the RBC membrane.
  - They have been associated with
    - Haemangiosarcoma (especially hepatic)
    - Glomerulonephritis
    - Lymphoma
    - Hepatic disease
- Heinz bodies (Figure 9.2)
  - Are round structure protruding from RBC membrane or a refractile spot in the cytoplasm

Table 9.1 Mechanisms and diseases associated with schistocytosis.

Shearing by fibrin strands:
• Microangiopathic haemolytic anaemia
• Disseminated intravascular coagulation
• Haemangiosarcoma
• Glomerulonephritis
• Myelofibrosis
• Haemolytic uremic syndrome
• Hypersplenism
Turbulent blood flow:
• Congestive heart failure
• Valvular stenosis
• Caval syndrome in heart worm disease
• Haemangiosarcoma
Intrinsic abnormalities:
• Chronic doxorubicin toxicosis
• Severe iron deficiency anaemia
• Pyruvate kinase deficiency
• Congenital and acquired dyserythropoiesis

- They are caused by oxidation, which results in denatured, precipitated haemoglobin
- They decrease RBC flexibility and therefore can cause intravascular haemolysis
- If removed by the spleen the may leave a spherocyte
- They are often found in small numbers in healthy cats but are almost always indicative of pathology in dogs
- Toxins that can cause oxidative injury include onion, garlic, paracetamol, excessive Vitamin K3, benzocaine-containing local anaesthetics, zinc and toilet bowl cleanser
- May also occur in splenectomised animals, after corticosteroid therapy and in patients with severe splenic dysfunction.

- Howell–Jolly bodies (Figure 9.1)
  - Are observed within the cytoplasm and are basophilic nuclear remnants
  - Their presence suggests regeneration or splenic dysfunction and can be normal in cats.

Diagnostic approach to acute or regenerative anaemia

Acute or regenerative anaemia can occur only in one of two ways – as a result of haemorrhage, haemolysis or occasionally both. Superficially, it might appear simple to differentiate haemorrhage from haemolysis as the cause of the anaemia, but often, differentiation poses a significant diagnostic dilemma.

Clues that can assist in deciding whether haemorrhage or haemolysis is present include the following:

- Clinical signs
  - Evidence for external haemorrhage?
  - Evidence for internal haemorrhage?
- Plasma protein concentration
- Autoagglutination present?
- Plasma appearance
  - Haemolysed?
- Degree of regeneration
- Urine
  - Haemoglobinuria?
  - Bilirubinuria?

Haemorrhage

If the haemorrhage is acute, there may initially be no change in the PCV, as both plasma and RBCs have been lost. However, after a few hours, the plasma will equilibrate, and the reduced PCV will become apparent.

Acute haemorrhage is often associated with decreased plasma protein concentrations, especially if the haemorrhage is external. If a patient has developed an acute anaemia and the plasma protein is high normal or above normal, then haemolysis is more likely than external haemorrhage. If there is evidence for external haemorrhage but the plasma protein is in the upper reference range or above, then consider that haemolysis may also be contributing to the anaemia.

Chronic external haemorrhage (e.g. gastroduodenal ulceration, bleeding GI tumour, intestinal parasites such as hookworms and severe flea infestation) will eventually cause iron deficiency, although the anaemia often remains moderately responsive. Anaemia due to chronic GI haemorrhage is usually associated with mild to moderate hypoproteinaemia. The platelet count is often high, normal or slightly elevated in chronic blood loss.

Internal haemorrhage into a body cavity may be difficult to detect, particularly intra-abdominal haemorrhage. With internal haemorrhage, the protein usually is less reduced than with external haemorrhage, because the protein is not 'lost' and plasma concentrations will increase more quickly after the bleed. Plasma concentrations will usually not be above normal, unless the patient is also dehydrated.

Intra-thoracic haemorrhage will usually cause acute, specific signs of compromised respiratory function. In contrast, intra-abdominal haemorrhage may be more difficult to identify. In particular, intra-abdominal haemorrhage is rapidly resorbed into the circulation (the peritoneum is a very large and efficient absorption surface), and thus, an acute splenic bleed of small to moderate volume, for example in a dog with haemangiosarcoma, may not be detectable by abdominocentesis within a few hours of the bleed.

Define the lesion

The key question when haemorrhage is detected is whether it is due to local disease (e.g. trauma and bleeding neoplasm) or systemic disease (e.g. coagulopathy and hypertension). This then permits the possible lesions to be defined – discussed in detail in Chapter 11.

Haemolysis

Anaemia resulting from haemolysis or internal haemorrhage tends to be more regenerative than that due to external blood loss, as all the iron is preserved and can be re-used. Haemolysis may occur extravascularly (RBCs are broken down in the reticuloendothelial system in the spleen predominantly, but also the liver and bone marrow) or intravascularly (RBCs are broken down within the bloodstream releasing haemoglobin). Increased serum bilirubin is observed in the majority (but not all) cases of extravascular haemolysis, although overt clinical jaundice may be less common. The diagnosis of haemolysis caused for example by IMHA should, therefore, never be excluded on the basis of the absence of overt jaundice.

Intravascular haemolysis can be easily demonstrated, as the plasma of a centrifuged (and appropriately collected) sample will be red if the intravascular haemolysis is moderate to severe. Haemoglobinuria is usually present in cases of intravascular haemolysis and jaundice is common. Differentiate from haematuria by centrifuging urine and observing the supernatant – it will be clear if haematuria is present and red if haemoglobinuria is present.

Regenerative anaemia

4 Define the lesion

Causes of haemolytic anaemia

Immune-mediated haemolytic anaemia (IMHA)

IMHA may be *primary* (idiopathic) or *secondary*, for example to drugs or neoplasia – particularly lymphoma. Primary (idiopathic) disease is most common in dogs. In the cat, IMHA is more frequently secondary to an underlying disease such as lymphoma or infectious disease. However, primary IMHA is being reported with increasing frequency in cats, although it is more commonly non-regenerative in this species.

Microangiopathic anaemia

Microangiopathic anaemia is a variant of haemolysis where the RBCs are physically damaged because they are forced through tortuous passages or are damaged by shearing forces (see Table 9.1).

Congenital haemolytic anaemia

Haemolytic anaemia may also occur in certain breeds with congenital defects of RBC metabolism, for example pyruvate kinase deficiency (Basenjis, West Highland White terriers) and phosphofructokinase deficiency (English Springer Spaniels who suffer acute, exercise-induced episodes of haemolysis). Usually, affected dogs have clinical signs from a relatively young age.

Infectious haemolytic anaemia

Mycoplasmosis or haemoplasmosis (infection usually with *Mycoplasma haemofelis*) is a potential cause of haemolytic anaemia in the cat. It should be noted that if a cat is positive for *M. haemofelis* but does not have a regenerative anaemia, other underlying disease should be sought. Older male non-pedigree cats are believed to be at increased risk for haemoplasma infection, although younger cats may be more likely to show signs of disease. The significance of infection is difficult to assess as asymptomatic carrier cats exist. Diagnosis should be made on the basis of PCR results (not blood smear alone) and should be interpreted in light of other clinical information. Anaemia due to *Mycoplasma* infection may be more likely in immunocompromised cats.

Babesiosis can cause haemolytic anaemia, which can mimic idiopathic IMHA. In endemic areas, it is often the most common cause of haemolytic anaemia. In non-endemic areas, the key question is travel history – if a dog has travelled outside a country such as the United Kingdom, then PCR testing for *Babesia* spp. is often appropriate.

Drug/toxins

Drugs such as sulphonamides, penicillin and methimazole have been associated with haemolytic anaemia, usually immune mediated. Paracetamol will cause haemolysis in cats, and zinc has been reported to cause severe haemolysis in both cats and dogs. Hypophosphataemia is a metabolic cause of haemolysis. History (drugs), biochemistry and plain radiography (zinc foreign body) can easily rule out these potential causes.

Non-regenerative anaemia

Define the lesion

Anaemia of chronic disease

Anaemia of chronic disease is the most common cause of non-regenerative anaemia. It is usually clinically innocuous and does not require treatment. However, it is an indication that there is an underlying disease present and warrants a vigorous search for its cause. It occurs with infectious, inflammatory or neoplastic disease. Anaemia of chronic disease is almost always normocytic, normochromic (if very prolonged microcytosis and hypochromasia can develop) and is usually mild (PCV 25–36% in dogs and 18–26% in cats). It should resolve if the underlying systemic disease is being treated successfully.

Chronic kidney disease

Anaemia is more likely with advanced stages of chronic kidney disease (CKD) (IRIS stages 3 and 4). It is simple to rule out by checking urea, creatinine and urine specific gravity.

Bone marrow disorders

Clues to bone marrow disease as a cause of non-regenerative anaemia include the following:

- RBCs are often normocytic and normochromic.
- The haemogram often contains major clues such as other cytopenia's, for example thrombocytopenia and neutropenia.
- Lymphopenia is relatively common and usually seen as part of a stress leukogram.
- If the animal has leukaemia or myelodysplasia, abnormal circulating cells may be seen on blood smear.

Bone marrow disorders include the following:

- Infection – parvovirus, panleukopenia and ehrlichiosis
- Toxic damage – oestrogen and chemotherapy
- Immune-mediated damage (pure red cell aplasia)
- Neoplasia – lymphoma, multiple myeloma, mast cell disease and leukaemias. Neoplastic cells compete for space and nutrients and release inhibitory factors. This is known as myelophthisis.
- Myelodysplasia – abnormal maturation or production of cells in the bone marrow
- Myelofibrosis – normal haemopoetic tissue is replaced by fibrous tissue. The cause of this is not always known.

Iron deficiency

Iron deficiency is a relatively uncommon cause of anaemia in small animals, but it can be overlooked as it doesn't tend to fit into the neat classification of regenerative or non-regenerative anaemia. It can be moderately regenerative to non-regenerative in nature. Fortunately, iron deficiency anaemia is fairly characteristic usually resulting in:

- Microcytosis (low MCV)
- Hypochromasia (low MCHC)
- Poikilocytosis
- Thrombocytosis if due to haemorrhage.

Iron deficiency in cats and early iron deficiency in dogs may be normocytic and normochromic. The most common cause of iron deficiency in adult small animals is chronic gastrointestinal blood loss.

In conclusion

The first step in assessing the patient with pale mucous membranes is to define the problem and system – decreased peripheral perfusion or anaemia? Once anaemia is confirmed, the most important thing to remember is that the numbers in a haemogram may not give you the whole picture. It is vitally important to assess RBC morphology to progress your understanding of the type of anaemia present and its possible causes. Always perform a smear and submit this to an external laboratory if you or your team does not have the confidence to adequately assess it in your practice.

CHAPTER 10
Jaundice

Jill E. Maddison
The Royal Veterinary College, Department of Clinical Science and Services, London, UK

Jaundice or icterus is a relatively common clinical sign. It is not often necessarily noted by owners and is usually detected by the veterinarian during their clinical examination of an unwell patient. It may also be observed in serum or identified in biochemistry results. The diagnostic approach to jaundice is straightforward, although confirming the final cause can be challenging.

1 Define the problem

Jaundice or icterus is a yellow discolouration of body tissues caused by increased levels of bilirubin. The normal liver has a large capacity to take up and excrete bilirubin. Therefore, jaundice will be observed clinically only when there is a large, persistent increase in bilirubin production or a major impairment in bilirubin excretion. The issue of defining the problem in relation to jaundice is not that it can be confused with another clinical sign but that it may be missed if the clinical examination is not sufficiently rigorous. Jaundice is most easily seen on sclera, mucous membranes and non-pigmented skin. Specific examination of the sclera during the clinical examination is important, as the sclera is not always obvious when observing an animal's face. Increased serum levels of bilirubin can be defined as a problem even if the animal isn't overtly jaundiced.

Physiology

Bilirubin is primarily formed from the breakdown of haemoglobin from aged red blood cells in the reticuloendothelial (RE) system of the spleen, liver, bone marrow and lymph nodes. A small amount is derived from myoglobin and heme-containing liver enzymes.

Clinical Reasoning in Small Animal Practice, First Edition.
Jill E. Maddison, Holger A. Volk and David B. Church.

Haemoglobin is split to release a protein molecule and heme (iron-containing porphyrin). The iron is released and stored in RE cells or re-used for heme synthesis. The remainder of heme is converted to biliverdin and then to bilirubin.

Bilirubin is transported to the liver in blood tightly bound to albumin – unconjugated bilirubin. Unconjugated bilirubin is not water soluble and is not filtered by the renal glomeruli or excreted by renal tubules.

Dogs (males more often than female) have a low resorptive threshold for bilirubin. They also have renal enzyme systems that produce and conjugate bilirubin to a limited extent. Therefore, mild bilirubinuria (up to 2+) can occur in normal dog urine with a specific gravity greater than 1.025. In contrast, cat kidneys cannot conjugate bilirubin, and their renal threshold is nine times higher than in dogs; therefore, bilirubinuria in a cat is always pathological.

In the liver, bilirubin is conjugated in hepatocytes and excreted into bile canaliculi and thence transported to the bile ducts and intestine.

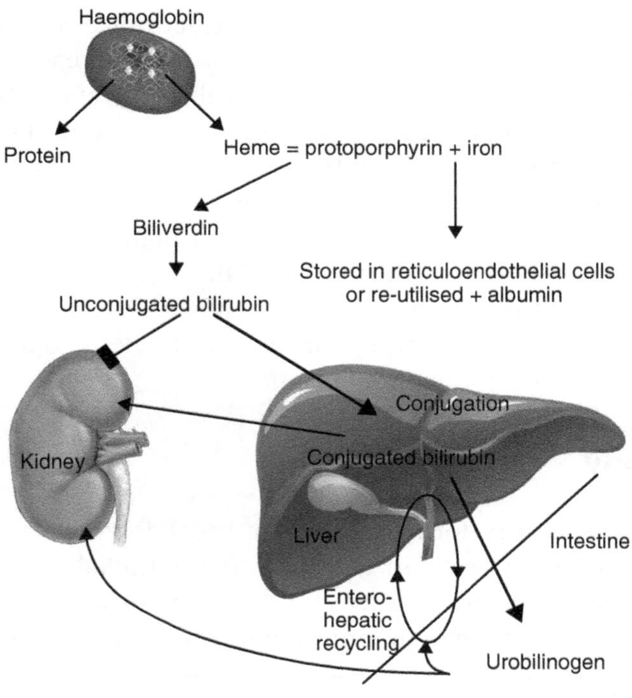

Figure 10.1 Bilirubin metabolism.

The excretion phase of bilirubin metabolism is the rate-limiting step in this process and will be overloaded first if there is excessive demand for bilirubin excretion.

Conjugated bilirubin is water soluble, dialysable and filtered by the kidneys – therefore, it can appear in urine. Conjugated bilirubin excreted through the bile duct into the small intestine is converted by colonic bacteria to urobilinogen (colourless), which is oxidised to urobilin (orange).

Some urobilinogen is reabsorbed by the intestine, enters the enterohepatic circulation and is re-excreted into the bile. A small amount is also excreted into urine (about 5%). Urobilinogen remaining in the intestinal tract is converted to stercobilinogen that is oxidized to stercobilin, which imparts normal faecal colour.

The metabolic pathway for bilirubin is illustrated in Figure 10.1.

Causes of jaundice

Define the system and location

The strict 'define the system then location approach' to problem solving theoretically is applicable to jaundice as a problem, but in practice, we tend to assess the system and location together. The system question relates to consideration of haematopoietic causes of jaundice vs. hepatobiliary causes, and this is the first key question. The combined system/location question relates to – 'is the jaundice due to pre-hepatic, hepatic or post-hepatic mechanisms?' It is relatively easier to differentiate haematopoietic from hepatobiliary causes but more challenging to differentiate hepatic from post-hepatic causes of jaundice.

Pre-hepatic jaundice

Pre-hepatic jaundice occurs when there is significant *red cell haemolysis*, which results in the bilirubin conjugation process in the liver being overwhelmed. Therefore, initially, primarily *unconjugated* bilirubin will be found in serum.

However, after a few days, there is also *conjugated* bilirubinaemia due to hepatic damage that occurs as a result of hypoxia and/or overloading of the excretory capacity of the hepatocytes. Thus, equal amounts of unconjugated and conjugated bilirubin will be found in the serum. Animals with red cell haemolysis that is severe enough to result in jaundice will *always have a significant anaemia*, which is usually regenerative assuming (i) that the bone marrow has had time to respond and (ii) that the patient doesn't have immune-mediated haemolytic anaemia with antibodies directed against RBC precursors as well as mature RBC.

Jaundice may also occur when there is significant internal (but not external) haemorrhage. Although the RBCs usually remain intact when blood is resorbed from the peritoneal cavity (autotransfusion), internal haemorrhage can result in RBC breakdown, which may overwhelm the capacity of the liver to take up, conjugate or secrete bilirubin. Jaundice is not a particularly common sequela of internal bleeding (although there may be slight increases in serum bilirubin on a biochemistry profile), but it should be considered in the anaemic patient, especially if they also have decreased plasma protein levels.

Define the lesion – pre-hepatic jaundice

Causes of haemolytic anaemia are discussed in detail in Chapter 9 and include the following:

- Immune-mediated haemolytic anaemia
- Microangiopathic haemolytic anaemia
- Congenital haemolytic anaemia
- Infectious causes
- Toxic causes
- Occasionally, internal haemorrhage causes haemolysis (see previous section).

Hepatic jaundice

Hepatic jaundice occurs with *hepatocellular disease*, which results in both conjugated (as the excretory capacity of liver is impaired) and unconjugated bilirubinaemia. There must be significant hepatocellular disease present before jaundice occurs. Jaundice is more likely to occur with hepatic disorders that involve primarily the periportal hepatocytes rather than centrilobular hepatocytes.

Define the lesion – hepatic jaundice

A liver biopsy is usually required to identify the type of hepatic pathology causing jaundice.

In dogs, hepatic causes of jaundice include cholangiohepatitis, leptospirosis and neoplasia, particularly lymphoma. Inflammatory liver disease tends not to cause jaundice as often in dogs as it does in cats. In dogs, the inflammatory process often involves the hepatic parenchyma, whereas in cats, it almost invariably involves the biliary system.

Cholangiohepatitis occurs more commonly in cats than in dogs and may be acute or chronic suppurative (neutrophillic) or non-suppurative (lymphocytic). Other hepatocellular diseases that may cause jaundice are feline infectious peritonitis (FIP) and neoplasia. Hepatic lipidosis is a relatively common cause of jaundice in North American cats but is uncommonly reported elsewhere, although there is evidence that the prevalence is increasing in some countries.

Post-hepatic jaundice

Post-hepatic jaundice occurs with *biliary tract disease*.

4 Define the lesion – post hepatic jaundice

Post-hepatic jaundice usually occurs with anatomic obstruction of bile ducts either within the liver or in the common bile duct.

Intra- or extra-hepatic bile duct obstruction can be due to a number of mechanisms, for example:

- toxic or infectious cholangitis
- pancreatic disease
  - for example, pancreatitis, pancreatic carcinoma, pancreatic abscess or pseudocyt
- infiltrating or space-occupying lesions (e.g. abscesses and neoplasms)
- cholelithiasis
- bile duct rupture
- obstruction of the bile duct at the level of its opening into the duodenum
  - for example, GI neoplasm or foreign body.

Abdominal ultrasound is a very useful diagnostic tool in confirming post-hepatic obstruction, although an exploratory laparotomy may be required to confirm the lesion. Bile duct rupture (traumatic or pathologic) will cause mild to moderate jaundice (depending on the time, cause and underlying pathology) and abdominal effusion. The bilirubin concentration in the abdominal effusion is usually greater than that of the serum. Bile is a very irritant fluid, and chemical peritonitis develops rapidly when bile leaks into the abdomen.

Non-hepatic causes of jaundice

Increased bilirubin levels may occur in patients with sepsis or severe inflammatory disease as inflammatory mediators interfere with bilirubin transport. Overt jaundice may be evident. This is particularly true in cats. Mild hyperbilirubinaemia (but not overt jaundice) may occur in a proportion of hyperthyroid cats. This may be due to increased degradation of hepatic heme proteins. Mild hyperbilirubinaemia (but not overt jaundice) may also occur with fever and starvation.

Differentiating causes of jaundice

Pre-hepatic

Pre-hepatic jaundice is easy to differentiate from hepatic and post-hepatic, as the animal will have a significant and regenerative anaemia. They may also have mild to moderately increased liver enzymes (possibly due to hypoxic damage), but the predominant feature is regenerative anaemia (without signs of haemorrhage – note that severe hepatocellular disease may cause coagulopathy).

Hepatic vs. post-hepatic

Hepatic and post-hepatic causes of jaundice are more difficult to differentiate. While an animal with only conjugated bilirubinaemia would most likely have post-hepatic jaundice, the majority of animals with hepatic or post-hepatic jaundice will have both unconjugated and conjugated bilirubinaemia. Post-hepatic obstruction will cause secondary hepatocellular damage, and as previously mentioned, bilirubin excretion is the first process to become disordered in primary hepatocellular disease.

Clinical signs

In some patients, the best clue to differentiation is the degree of malaise the animal presents with. In general (there are *always* exceptions), if an animal is jaundiced but relatively well, it most probably has post-hepatic disease. Primary hepatocellular disorders of sufficient severity to cause jaundice are usually accompanied by marked clinical signs of liver disease. However, animals with both hepatic and post-hepatic disease can obviously present extremely unwell, depending on the underlying aetiology.

Serum enzymology

Serum enzymology (alanine aminotransferase, ALT; alkaline phosphatase, ALP) is also not often helpful in differentiating hepatic and post-hepatic jaundice. Post-hepatic obstruction almost invariably causes secondary hepatocellular damage, and hence, both ALT and ALP will be elevated. ALP is elevated by both intra- and extra-hepatic cholestasis, thus is increased in hepatic and post-hepatic disease. However, if the ALT is substantially elevated (over 1000 U/L) and the ALP is only slightly or moderately elevated (<500 U/L), this suggests hepatic parenchymal pathology.

Serum bile acids

Serum bile acids are useful in confirming the presence of liver disease when other test results are equivocal. However, in a jaundiced animal, once you have ruled out pre-hepatic causes (based on the haemogram) and sepsis (based on the white blood cell count and other clinical signs), bile acids will not assist in differentiating hepatic from post-hepatic disease and will not give you any further information about the type of liver disease present.

Bile acid excretion is not related to or affected by bilirubin excretion. Bile acids, therefore, can be useful in assessing the liver in a patient whose jaundice is due to haemolysis (i.e. pre-hepatic), and they may also be useful to assess the liver if a non-hepatic septic/inflammatory cause of jaundice is being considered.

Diagnostic imaging

Hepatic ultrasound is a useful tool in differentiating hepatic from post-hepatic causes of jaundice, as it will reveal whether the bile duct is obstructed and dilated and whether there are diffuse changes in the liver parenchyma. However, ultrasound cannot define the type of tissue pathology in many cases (inflammatory vs. infectious, neoplastic vs. toxic etc.). Plain radiographs are usually unhelpful in differentiating hepatic from post-hepatic causes of jaundice.

Non-hepatic

Non-hepatic septic or severe inflammatory disorders causing jaundice (bilirubin usually <50 μmol/L) will usually be associated with other clinical and clinical pathology signs of inflammation, although this is not invariable. If the bilirubin level is greater than 50 μmol/L, an hepatobiliary cause is almost certainly present (assuming the patient is not anaemic). But if the level is less than 50 μmol/L, the patient is pyrexic and/or has an inflammatory leukogram; don't assume that the location of the lesion must be the hepatobiliary system.

Why is it important to differentiate hepatic from post-hepatic causes of jaundice?

The reason why it is important to determine whether the animal has post-hepatic obstruction rather than primary hepatocellular disease is that surgical correction of post-hepatic obstruction *may* be feasible, whereas surgery is usually indicated in primary hepatocellular disease to obtain biopsies. Hepatic biopsies may be obtainable by other means (such as ultrasound-guided percutaneous biopsy or laparoscopy).

The surgical expertise required to correct post-hepatic obstructions can be considerable, and it is important to recognise that a specialist surgeon may be needed if your own surgical skills do not extend to procedures such as cholecystojejunostomy.

In conclusion

Jaundice is a clinical problem that may be detected on clinical examination or by laboratory testing. It almost always indicates serious pathology, the location of which can be the haematopoietic system (haemolysis), liver, the biliary tract or peri-hepatobiliary structures such as the pancreas. It can also be caused by severe inflammation and sepsis. A rational approach involves appreciation of the relevant pathophysiology, as well as recognition that differentiating hepatic from post-hepatic causes can be challenging and often requires a multi-modal diagnostic approach.

CHAPTER 11

Bleeding

Jill E. Maddison
The Royal Veterinary College, Department of Clinical Science and Services, London, UK

Bleeding is a potentially life-threatening clinical sign, which often requires prompt assessment and management. As with all clinical signs, a structured approach is the key to ensuring that important differentials are not overlooked. Understanding the pathophysiology of bleeding is also important, particularly in relation to interpreting relevant clinical pathology. Three major bleeding sites are discussed in this chapter, but the principles of the approach apply to any site of bleeding – most importantly – is this animal bleeding because of local disease or systemic disease?

Diagnostic approach to the bleeding patient

1 Define the problem

The potential for confusing bleeding as a clinical sign with another clinical sign is variable dependent on the site of bleeding. The issue can be 'is this *blood*'? (e.g. red urine), or 'is the cause *pathological*?' (e.g. melaena).

Epistaxis

Epistaxis is defined as bleeding from the nose. It is unlikely that identification of the problem will pose any difficulties, although confirming the blood is coming from within the nasal cavity as opposed to perinasal skin is important (the latter almost always due to local trauma or skin pathology).

Melaena

Melaena is the presence of digested blood in the faeces and is manifested as black tarry faeces. It can also be detected using tests for occult

Clinical Reasoning in Small Animal Practice, First Edition.
Jill E. Maddison, Holger A. Volk and David B. Church.

faecal blood. It is important to determine whether the melaena is due only to the animal having eaten a very high meat meal (therefore, obtaining a dietary history is important) or has swallowed blood – that is, is bleeding in the mouth or nasal cavity, coughing up blood then swallowing it or licking a bleeding wound.

Red urine

Red urine may be due to haematuria, haemoglobinuria, myoglobinuria or even ingestion of beetroot (beeturia). Hence, for the animal presenting with what the owner describes as 'blood in the urine', an important first step is to confirm that the urine discolouration is in fact due to the presence of red blood cells.

Clinical signs may assist (see the following sections) or a simple method is to spin some urine down and examine the sediment and supernatant. In cases of 'pseudohaematuria', the supernatant will remain discoloured. Urine dipsticks cannot differentiate between lysed blood cells, 'pure' haemoglobin and myoglobin.

Define the system

Any site of bleeding such as epistaxis, melaena and haematuria may be due to local disorders or systemic disorders – this is the key question to answer, which has a profound impact on the diagnostic pathway and potential differentials. Systemic disorders include bleeding disorders (coagulopathy), hypertension, polycythaemia, hyperviscosity and systemic vasculitis.

Define the lesion

We will first consider local disorders for the specific signs and then the diagnostic approach to bleeding disorders in general.

Local disorders

Epistaxis

Local disorders that can cause epistaxis include the following:

- Neoplasia

- Inflammatory/infectious
  - Immune-mediated or allergic rhinitis
  - Fungal infection
  - Local vasculitis
- Severe dental disease, for example, tooth root abscess
- Trauma
- Foreign bodies.

Clues

The diagnostic approach to local disorders or systemic disorders is obviously very different; thus, the initial goal should be to try to identify clues from the physical examination and history that suggest whether local or systemic disease is present.

Site of bleeding

Careful examination for any signs of bleeding at other sites (mucous membranes, skin, haematuria, melaena and retina) is essential. Whether the epistaxis is unilateral or bilateral may also be helpful – a bleeding disorder is less likely to cause a unilateral discharge, although this is by no means an absolute finding.

Character of the nasal discharge

Neoplasia, fungal infections and foreign bodies will often cause a mucopurulent, as well as haemorrhagic nasal discharge. The animal may have a history of sneezing (more likely with local nasal lesions than bleeding disorders, but sneezing can still occur with systemic causes).

Nasal examination

Local disorders causing epistaxis may be associated with swelling or deformity along the nasal cavity, ulceration of the nares (fungal disease) and/or evidence of disruption/displacement of the nasal septum on radiographs.

If the animal has only epistaxis with no mucopurulent component, no signs of swelling or pain and no history of sneezing, a bleeding disorder should be considered even if there is no other site of haemorrhage detected (unusual).

Local disorders – diagnostic approach

If a local disorder is suspected and the patient cannot be referred for computed tomography (CT) (see the following sections and Chapter 8), the diagnostic approach should involve nasal biopsies via aggressive intranasal aspiration and washings, radiography (maxillary views – 'radiographic plate in the mouth' technique) and/or rhinoscopy if the equipment is available. Note that haemorrhagic/mucopurulent nasal discharge may occur with severe dental disease, so this should obviously be excluded as a cause before embarking on intranasal investigations.

Exploratory surgery of the nasal cavity is a messy and invasive procedure, and it is prudent to avoid it if possible. The following guidelines pertinent to local nasal disorders apply:

1 Fungal and neoplastic causes of epistaxis are relatively common. Aspergillosis is the most common fungal disease observed in various countries; neoplasia includes adenocarcinoma, squamous cell carcinoma, lymphosarcoma, fibrosarcoma, chrondosarcoma, haemangiosarcoma and osteosarcoma.
2 Nasal biopsy/washings are best performed with some type of relatively rigid catheter, which is forcefully inserted into the nasal cavity as far as possible. Measure externally the length from the nares to the frontal sinus – cut a large stiff urinary catheter to this length (or mark it) and insert. Forceful aspiration is mandatory – gentle nasal washings with saline are usually unrewarding.
3 Radiology is often of value if you can obtain radiographs of the maxilla only, that is intra-oral radiograph or ventrodorsal open mouth views. Both neoplasia and fungal disease will cause turbinate and septum destruction, but septal deviation is usually only caused by neoplasia.
4 CT scanning is an extremely useful diagnostic tool in the diagnostic work up of the patient with epistaxis due to local disease and should be considered as a diagnostic option if at all possible ahead of the previously mentioned procedures.

Melaena

Melaena can occur due to gastrointestinal (GI) ulceration or due to bleeding disorders. In the latter case, there is no overt ulceration, and the use of anti-ulcer drugs in the management of these cases is not indicated.

Melaena due to GI ulceration may occur due to primary GI disease (neoplasia, parasites such as hookworms and foreign bodies) or secondary GI diseases that cause ulceration (e.g. liver disease, mast cell tumours, gastrinoma, NSAID toxicity and hypoadrenocorticism). It is therefore important that you do not immediately assume that the presence of melaena indicates primary GI disease, even if vomiting is also present, as many of the secondary GI causes of ulceration will also cause vomiting (see Chapter 2). Failure to recognise this may result in very inappropriate diagnostic procedures (e.g. endoscopy) being performed.

Haematuria

Haematuria is most commonly due to local disease but, similarly to other sites of bleeding, can occur as a consequence of systemic disease.

Local disorders

The causes of haematuria due to local disease include the following:

- Urinary calculi
- Neoplasia
  - bladder neoplasia (most commonly transitional cell carcinoma)
  - neoplasia of the renal pelvis
  - polyps
- Inflammatory/infectious
  - bacterial cystitis
  - prostatitis
  - interstitial cystitis (cats)
- Idiopathic
  - idiopathic renal haemorrhage
- Vascular anomalies.

Clues

Inflammatory lower urinary tract disease is usually associated with dysuria and/or pollakiuria. If the animal has haematuria without signs of pollakiuria or dysuria, then renal or ureteral haemorrhage (from any cause), cystic neoplasia, polyps or a systemic bleeding disorder should be considered.

The location of the bleeding in relation to the process of micturition may give some clues.

- If bleeding occurs at the beginning of urination, disorders of the lower urogenital tract – bladder neck, urethra, prostate, vagina, vulva, penis or prepuce – should be considered.
- Dogs with prostatitis will often drip blood unrelated to urination.
- Blood occurring at the end of urination or throughout urination is usually due to upper urinary tract disorders – bladder, ureters or kidneys.

Diagnostic approach

Identification of the cause of haematuria due to local disorders usually requires urinalysis +/− culture and sensitivity +/− diagnostic imaging. If a lesion has not been identified by these methods and a bleeding disorder has been ruled out (see the following sections), exploratory surgery may be required.

Systemic bleeding disorders

Diagnosis and understanding of systemic bleeding disorders require an understanding of the normal process of coagulation.

When a vessel wall is damaged, a number of processes come into play to attempt to heal the vascular damage. The factors involved in forming a haemostatic plug are interdependent, and a defect at any level can result in a bleeding disorder.

Classically, three systems (the vascular wall, the primary haemostatic system and the secondary haemostatic system) are considered to be responsible for healing vascular damage. This classical approach to the coagulation system forms a basis for understanding many of the commonly used clinical coagulation tests. However, the classical approach does not explain all of the clinically observed findings relating to coagulation abnormalities (such as the observation that Factor XII deficiency is not clinically significant, whereas Factor VII deficiency results in a severe coagulopathy), and this has resulted in the development of an alternative or 'cell-based' model of coagulation. The reader is referred to other texts if they wish to delve more deeply into this area of physiology and pathophysiology.

As Figure 11.1 demonstrates, vessel wall function, platelet function and the coagulation cascade are all involved in the formation

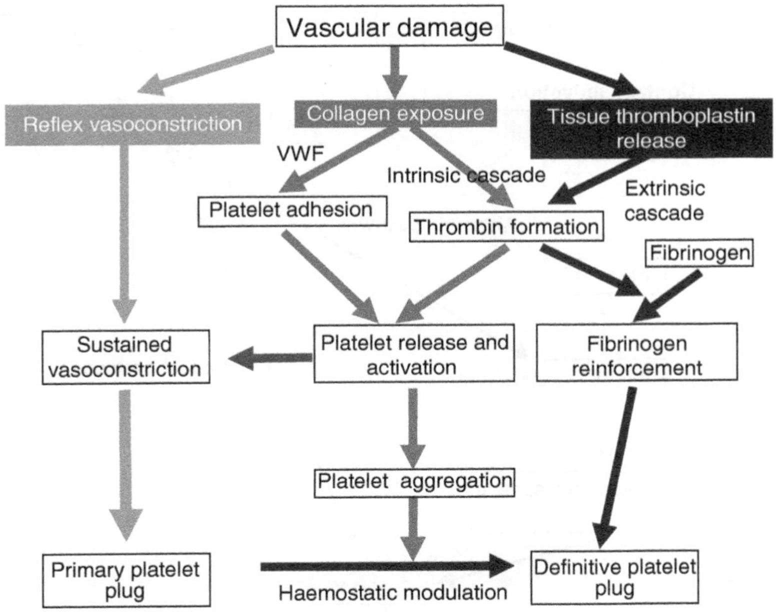

Figure 11.1 Formation of the definitive platelet plug.

of a primary haemostatic plug after vascular damage has occurred. Figure 11.2 shows the classical coagulation cascade.

Causes of haemorrhage

Bleeding may occur if there is:

- An abnormality of the *vessel wall*
  - trauma
  - vasculitis
- Reduced *platelet numbers*
  - thrombocytopenia
- *Platelet dysfunction*
  - lack of von Willebrand's factor – vWF
  - defect in activation and aggregation
- A defect in the extrinsic or intrinsic *coagulation cascade*
  - Haemophilia A and B
  - Vitamin K disorders
  - Disseminated intravascular coagulation (DIC).

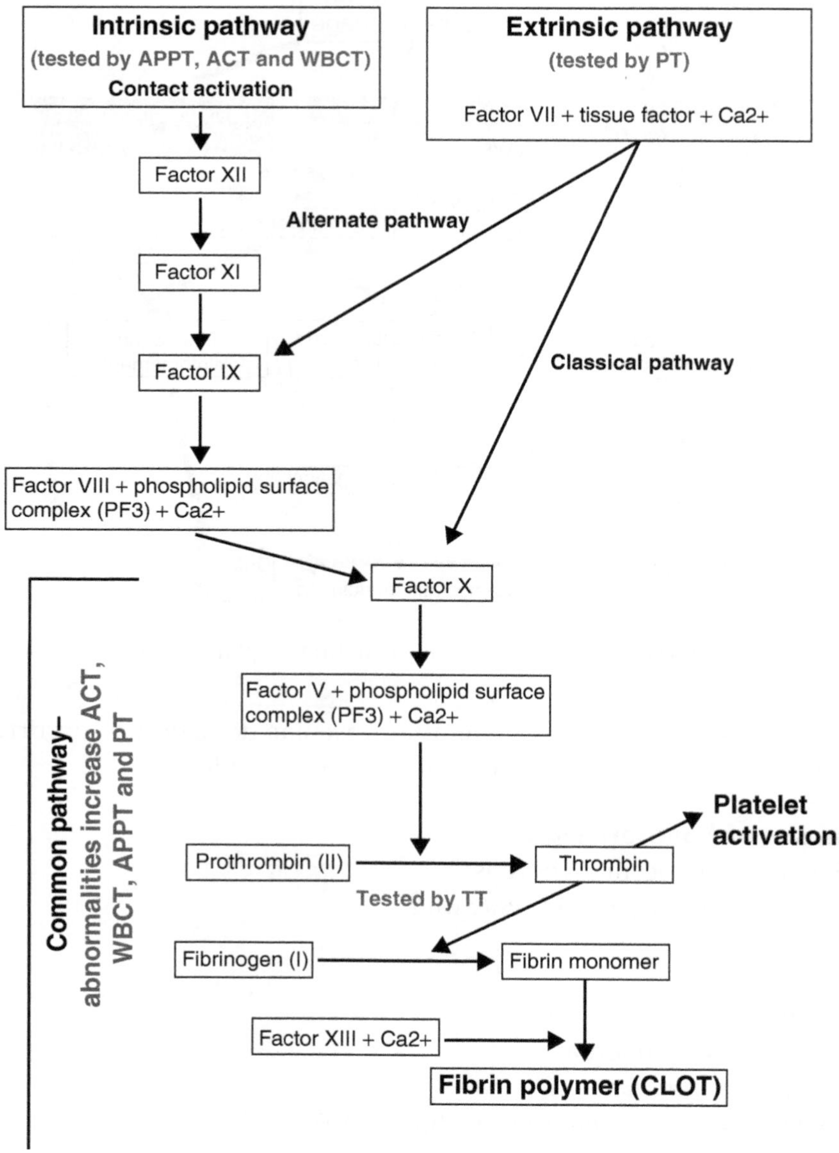

Figure 11.2 The coagulation cascade.

Table 11.1 Changes in coagulation tests associated with bleeding disorders.

Bleeding disorder	Coagulation tests results
Disorders of the intrinsic coagulation pathway (*e.g. Haemophilia A*)	• Prolonged activated clotting time (ACT) • Prolonged whole blood clotting time (WBCT) • Prolonged activated partial thromboplastin time (APTT) • Normal prothrombin time (PT)
Disorders of the extrinsic pathway (*e.g. Haemophilia B*)	• Prolonged PT • Normal APTT
Disorders of the common pathway or multifactor disorders • Hereditary common pathway defects (*factor II or X deficiency*) • Acquired multiple factor deficiencies (*DIC, liver disease*) • Vitamin K disorders (*warfarin toxicity, malabsorption of vitamin K, liver disease, Devon Rex coagulopathy*)	• Prolonged WBCT • Prolonged ACT • Prolonged PT • Prolonged APTT • Thrombin time (TT) will also be abnormal in DIC and fibrin degradation products will be reported
von Willebrand's disease	• WBCT, ACT, PT, APTT and TT will usually be normal • Buccal mucosal bleeding time and clot retraction will be prolonged
Acquired or congenital platelet dysfuction	• Buccal mucosal bleeding time and clot retraction will be prolonged

In addition, disorders such as hypertension and hyperviscosity will increase the tendency for exudation to occur and will perturb platelet function.

Diagnosis of bleeding disorders

The changes in coagulation tests that occur with different bleeding disorders are summarized in Table 11.1.

Clinical signs

- Reduced platelet numbers or impaired platelet function usually manifests as bleeding from mucosal surfaces, for example petechiation.

- In contrast, clotting factor deficiencies (from any cause) usually manifest as deeper tissue (ecchymosis) and body cavity haemorrhages.
- Petechiation can also occur with vasculitis.

Platelet count

The first test is a platelet count. Ensure that you specifically request a platelet count from your laboratory if you are investigating a bleeding disorder, as many laboratories assess platelet numbers only qualitatively unless specifically requested.

Although in-house haematology machines may be useful, they may also be inaccurate, and clinicians should be familiar with the assessment of platelet counts on a fresh blood smear. Generally 8–15 platelets per high power field (×100) would be considered normal. Clinical bleeding is unlikely unless the platelet count drops below 50×10^9/L (usually $<30 \times 10^9$/L), which is approximately 3–4 platelets per high power field. The presence of multiple platelet clumps in the feathered edge is likely to represent numbers adequate for haemostasis.

Buccal mucosal bleeding time

Buccal mucosal bleeding time can be measured easily but does require a standard cut being made in the buccal mucosa and strict attention to detail when timing the formation of a clot. This is usually performed using a commercial device such as the Surgicutt® on the buccal mucosa. Two to four minutes is considered normal. The buccal mucosal bleeding time is a crude screening test for platelet abnormalities. In animals with platelet dysfunction (e.g. von Willebrand's disease), it will often be the only readily available test that can confirm that a tendency to bleed is present.

Whole blood clotting time

Whole blood clotting time (WBCT) is a crude measure of the function of the intrinsic and common pathways. The glass surface acts as an initiator of intrinsic coagulation, and the phospholipid required is provided by platelets.

Place 1–2 mL of blood into a glass test tube (with a stopper) and invert tube every 30 seconds. Complete clot formation occurs when the blood ceases to flow up the tube. Plastic is a very poor activator of clotting, and therefore, containers such as plastic syringes should not be used to assess the WBCT.

WBCT in normal dogs at room temperature is 6.1 ± 0.2 minutes. WBCT will increase with defects in the intrinsic and common pathways and with *severe* thrombocytopenia.

Activated clotting time

The activated clotting time (ACT) test involves placing 2 mL of whole blood into a tube containing diatomaceous earth, an inert surface activating agent. An abnormal ACT indicates a defect in the coagulation cascade, specifically the intrinsic and common pathways. The ACT does not assess platelet number or function; however, as traces of platelet factor 3 are essential for activation of the clotting cascade, the ACT may be prolonged in the presence of severe thrombocytopenia ($<10 \times 10^9$/L).

The ACT is more reproducible at body temperature (38°C) than at room temperature. Therefore, ACT testing is performed optimally using a block heater or water bath or, if these are not available, by holding the tube within cupped hands.

A prolonged ACT suggests the presence of a severe coagulopathy. As the ACT is a relatively insensitive screening test, it may miss patients with mildly defective secondary haemostasis. The activated partial thromboplastin time (APTT) (see the following section) evaluates the same clotting pathways as the ACT but is more sensitive. Therefore, it is possible for a patient to have a normal ACT but a prolonged APTT.

Activated partial thromboplastin time

APTT assesses the *intrinsic* coagulation and common pathways. It is performed by incubating citrated blood with an activator of factor XII (kaolin or celite) and cephaloplastins, which substitute for platelet phospholipid requirements. After the addition of ionic calcium, the time taken to form fibrin is measured. In factor-deficient states, there must be at least a 30% deficiency of a factor before the APTT is increased.

Prothrombin time

Measurement of the one-stage prothrombin time assesses the *extrinsic* coagulation pathway. A thromboplastin–calcium mixture is added to citrated plasma, and the time taken to form fibrin is measured. Phospholipids in the thromboplastin mixture make the test independent of platelet function. The PT is very sensitive to warfarin toxicity or vitamin K deficiency due to the short half-life of factor VII.

Thrombin time

The thrombin time (TT) measures the reactivity of fibrinogen to exogenous thrombin. It is independent of the intrinsic and extrinsic coagulation pathways. TT is prolonged in conditions causing hypofibrinogenaemia (DIC, liver disease) or dysfibrinogenaemia (liver disease). The TT may also be prolonged by thrombin inhibitors such as fibrin degradation products and heparin.

von Willebrand's factor

vWF is measured in citrated plasma, which has been frozen in plastic tubes after immediate separation from red blood cells. The test is an ELISA assay.

Platelet function

Platelet function can be assessed by various methods including clot retraction – a relatively simple test that can be performed in commercial laboratories.

A crude measure of platelet function that can be performed in-house is as follows: place a sample of blood into a glass test tube and leave it to stand for 4–6 hours. Clot retraction can be calculated by measuring the height of the clot compared to the height of the total sample in the tube. The clot should separate from the serum and contract to approximately 50% of the original volume by 4–6 hours. Clot retraction will be reduced if there is platelet dysfunction or if there is a significant thrombocytopenia (hence, the test is mainly useful once thrombocytopenia has been ruled out as a cause of the coagulopathy).

Quality control

Various factors can interfere with coagulation tests. Excitement can increase platelet counts, increase platelet aggregation and increase levels of factor V, factor VIII, vWF and fibrinogen.

Samples collected for coagulation tests are usually collected into citrated tubes at a ratio of 1 part sodium citrate to 9 parts blood.

Either plastic tubes or siliconised glass tubes may be used (note that most glass collecting tubes are not siliconised). For the measurement of vWF, plasma should be harvested after centrifugation using plastic pipettes or syringes and plasma stored in plastic tubes.

Excessive sodium citrate will cause a prolongation of tests due to decreased calcium causing a delayed fibrin clot. Polycythaemia causes plasma to be overcitrated if the 1:9 ratio is used. More importantly, if the 1:9 ratio is used on anaemic blood, the plasma will be undercitrated – discuss with your laboratory how to compensate for these problems.

In general, prolongation of clotting times is regarded as significant if the patient time is more than 33% greater than the control sample. When using reference ranges, remember that 5% of the normal population will fall outside of the reference range (as the range is mean ±2 SD), so interpret with great care results that are only a few seconds outside the reference range. Decreased clotting times are not clinically relevant.

Causes of bleeding disorders

The most common causes of impaired coagulation are as follows:

- Immune-mediated thrombocytopenia (ITP)
- von Willebrand's disease
- Drug-induced platelet dysfunction
- Rodenticide poisoning
- DIC
- *Angiostrongylus vasorum* infection (in endemic areas).

Other less common causes include the following:

- Inherited platelet dysfunction
- Inherited coagulation factor deficiencies
- Malabsorption of vitamin K
- Acquired disorders of platelet function.

Thrombocytopenia

Thrombocytopenia may occur due to:

- Inadequate *production* of platelets
- Excessive *consumption* of platelets
- Excessive *destruction* of platelets
- *Infectious* causes (often a combination of mechanisms).

Unless there is a concurrent platelet function defect, haemorrhage due to thrombocytopenia will usually not occur until the platelet count is well below normal, usually at or below 30×10^9 cells/L (normal range $200–400 \times 10^9$ cells/L). As acute haemorrhage can cause moderate to marked thrombocytopenia, moderately sub-normal platelet counts should not be over-interpreted, as they may be a consequence rather than a cause of haemorrhage. Platelet numbers are rarely reduced below 50×10^9 cells/L as a result of haemorrhage alone.

Inadequate production

Inadequate production of platelets by the bone marrow is associated with:

- *Primary bone marrow disorders* such as myelophthisis (replacement of blood-forming cells by neoplastic or inflammatory tissue).
- *Drugs* such as oestrogen and cytotoxic agents may suppress platelet production. Various other drugs can also cause thrombocytopenia – many also cause anaemia and/or neutropenia. In general, thrombocytopenia due to bone marrow failure will be associated with depression of other blood-forming cells. An exception is the haemogram seen in the early stages of oestrogen toxicity when a neutrophilia is usually observed (neutropenia develops later). Endogenous oestrogen toxicity due to testicular or ovarian tumours causing thrombocytopenia has been reported but is rare.
- Retroviral infections (FeLV, FIV) in cats can cause thrombocytopenia and should be considered in a thrombocytopenic cat with no history of previous medication.

Excessive destruction

Excessive destruction of platelets is usually a result of immune-mediated processes. ITP is the most common cause of thrombocytopenia in dogs but is rare in cats. ITP can be a primary autoimmune disorder, induced by live vaccines or drugs or secondary to underlying pathology such as neoplasia. Endotoxaemia and sepsis can also cause excessive destruction of platelets.

Definitive diagnosis of ITP can be difficult and requires a platelet factor 3 test (not widely available and often negative anyway), measurement of anti-platelet antibodies (not widely available) and/or a bone marrow examination (reveals 'maturation arrest' of megakaryocytes). However, at least in dogs, if oestrogen toxicity can be ruled out from the history, there is no prior history of drug administration or vaccination that could cause thrombocytopenia, there is no evidence of underlying disease that might cause DIC (or it is ruled out by normal coagulation tests), infectious causes are ruled out due to geography and the platelet count is sufficiently low to cause haemorrhage ($<30 \times 10^9$); a diagnosis of ITP can usually be made from the haemogram alone. In cats, FeLV and FIV infection and other causes of decreased platelet production should be thoroughly investigated, as immune mediated platelet destruction is a rare cause of thrombocytopenia.

Excessive consumption

Excessive consumption of platelets occurs in DIC. DIC occurs as a result of intravascular activation of coagulation together with fibrinolysis. As a result, thrombosis occurs in multiple organs, platelets and coagulation factors are consumed and become depleted and fibrin degradation products (FDPs) interfere with platelet function.

Excessive consumption or sequestration can also occur in microangiopathy (this should also be associated with haemolytic anaemia).

Infectious causes

Tick-borne disease such as canine erlichiosis, Rocky Mountain spotted fever, cyclic thrombocytopenia, anaplasmosis and babesiosis can all cause thrombocytopenia and should be considered if these diseases are endemic to the area or the patient has travelled to endemic areas.

The bleeding diathesis that can occur in a proportion of dogs with *Angiostrongylus vasorum* infection can be associated with a variety of coagulation abnormalities including thrombocytopenia. The mechanism of coagulopathy is currently unknown – a form of chronic DIC seems to be the most likely explanation, although reports exist of severe thrombocytopenia and acquired von Willebrand's disease in association with angiostrongylosis. Successful treatment of the parasite will result in resolution of the coagulopathy.

Miscellaneous causes

Rare causes of clinically significant thrombocytopenia due to consumption and/or sequestration and/or destruction of platelets include haemolytic uraemic syndrome, thrombotic thrombocytopenia purpura, endotoxaemia, vasculitis, splenomegaly, splenic torsion and acute hepatic necrosis.

In conclusion

As with many other clinical signs, the assessment of the bleeding patient requires a structured approach. This must be underpinned by appreciation of pathophysiology so that the results of diagnostic tests can be appropriately assessed. The very first step when faced with a bleeding patient is to define the system – is the bleeding due to local or systemic disease? The answer can be obvious or require investigation, but the aim is to avoid a serious clinical error by neglecting to ensure that coagulation is normal before proceeding with invasive diagnostic tests to assess local disease such as biopsy.

CHAPTER 12
Polyuria/polydipsia and/or impaired urine concentration

Jill E. Maddison[1] & David B. Church[2]
[1]The Royal Veterinary College, Department of Clinical Science and Services, London, UK
[2]The Royal Veterinary College, London, UK

Polyuria/polydipsia (PU/PD) is a relatively frequent presenting complaint in small animal practice. A wide range of disorders ranging from clinically inconsequential to life threatening may cause polydipsia and/or polyuria, and an ordered, rational diagnostic approach to the problem, as well as an understanding of the underlying pathophysiological processes, is invaluable in the successful investigation and management of these cases. Polyuric disorders may also be recognised when impaired urine concentration is identified during case assessment. We will discuss the pathophysiology of PU/PD first and then move to discussing a structured diagnostic approach.

Pathophysiology

Classifying the mechanisms of polyuria/polydipsia

Polydipsia and polyuria can really occur only for two basic reasons – either the animal is drinking too much water and thus has polyuria as a *normal* consequence of increased water intake or it has impaired renal concentrating capacity resulting in increased urine volume and thus increased water intake to maintain neutral water balance.

When the cause is an increase in water intake, the problem can be categorised as *primary polydipsia*. Although a number of well-defined endocrine disorders can result in primary polydipsia, most patients with this problem are otherwise unremarkable in every other way. Effectively, this is a behavioural abnormality or a

Clinical Reasoning in Small Animal Practice, First Edition.
Jill E. Maddison, Holger A. Volk and David B. Church.

form of cerebrocortical dysfunction and can be thought of as either a primary (intra-cranial) or a secondary (extra-cranial) abnormality (see Chapter 7).

If the polydipsia occurs to compensate for increased urine production, then clearly, this is a result of impaired renal concentrating ability. The concentrating ability of the kidney is dependent on a number of factors, and each of these can result in increased urine volume and thus consequently polydipsia.

Reduced nephron number and function

Creation of a highly concentrated renal interstitum with a gradient of increasing concentration from renal cortex to renal medulla is essential for the formation of concentrated urine. The creation and maintenance of this gradient is dependent upon *normal numbers* of *normally functioning* nephrons. Consequently, reduced nephron function results in a diminished concentration gradient within the renal interstitium and impaired capacity to modify tubular filtrate and hence urine concentration.

Disorders that result in markedly reduced numbers of nephrons, or where nephron numbers are normal but their ability to create the concentrated renal interstitium is impaired, will result in increased urine volume and polydipsia.

Impaired antidiuretic hormone function

The second mechanism resulting in an impaired ability to concentrate the urine and thus polydipsia occurs when the renal interstitial concentration gradient is normal but the part of the nephron responsible for water moving from the tubular filtrate down its concentration gradient to the concentrated interstitium (the collecting tubule) remains impermeable to water. The permeability of the collecting duct to water and urea is a direct result of antidiuretic hormone (ADH) binding to its receptors on the collecting tubules. When this process is impaired, it is caused by a primary ADH deficiency or systemic factors interfering with ADH's binding to or activation of its receptors.

Altered osmolarity of the glomerular filtrate

The third means by which urine concentrating mechanisms can be impaired has nothing to do with modifications of the kidney itself but occurs when the tubular filtrate itself contains greater than normal numbers of osmotically active particles. When this occurs, the osmotic gradient between the tubular filtrate and the renal interstitium is reduced, and a diminished volume of water can be withdrawn from the tubular filtrate, even though both the renal interstitial osmotic gradient and the permeability of the collecting tubule are completely normal.

Summary

As can be seen from the aforementioned descriptions, the mechanisms that result in PU/PD can be classified according to the particular pathophysiological process resulting in either increased water intake or the various reasons for impaired capacity to concentrate the tubular filtrate.

Thus, PU/PD can be due to:

1 *Primary polydipsia*. Some of the disorders that can produce PU/PD through this mechanism include the following:
   - Psychogenic causes
   - Hyperadrenocorticism (part of the explanation – may also cause impaired urine concentration)
   - Hepatic encephalopathy (part of the explanation – may also cause impaired urine concentration)
   - Hyperthyroidism
   - Hypothalamic lesion affecting thirst receptors (rare)
   - Drug effect on thirst centre (e.g. phenobarbitone)

2 *Structural renal tubule damage resulting in reduced medullary hypertonicity*. The disorders most likely to result in PU/PD through this mechanism include the following:
   - Chronic kidney disease (CKD)
   - Pyelonephritis
   - Nephrocalcinosis

3 *Impaired nephron function resulting in reduced medullary hypertonicity*. The disorders most likely to result in PU/PD through this mechanism include the following:
   - Hyponatraemia
     - Hypoadrenocorticism
     - Profound gut sodium loss

Table 12.1 Pathophysiology of PU/PD.

Disorder	Pathophysiology
Psychogenic polydipsia	Psychogenic polydipsia is a behavioural disorders causing primary polydipsia, which causes compensatory (and appropriate) polyuria. The cause is unknown but it is speculated that anxiety may be a cause in some animals.
Hyperadrenocorticism	The mechanism by which hyperadrenocorticism causes PU/PD in dogs is not well understood. It is thought that cortisol may interfere with ADH function. However, frequently, dogs with hyperadrenocorticism can reduce their water intake and urine output when initially hospitalised, which would suggest that other factors are important. PU/PD does not occur in humans with hyperadrenocorticism or in humans on corticosteroid medication, which is a fascinating species difference. Clinical impressions are that cats become polydipsic after corticosteroid treatment much less frequently than dogs, which also suggests an interesting species difference.
Hepatic disease	The mechanism by which hepatic disease, especially portosystemic encephalopathy, causes polyuria is also unknown. Various theories have been proposed – decreased urea concentration in the medullary interstitium may be a factor. However, some dogs with portosystemic shunts can concentrate their urine when challenged, whereas others can't. It is possible that the polydipsia, rather than the polyuria, may be primary and a neurobehavioral consequence of encephalopathy.
Hyperthyroidism	The mechanism by which hyperthyroidism causes PU/PD is multifactorial. Thyroxine increases effective renal blood flow due to dilation of the pre-glomerular arterial vessel, which causes increased GFR and hyperfiltration. It has been suggested that increased renal blood flow may also impair urine-concentrating ability by causing medullary solute washout. It is also possible that thyrotoxicosis produces a primary, compulsive polydipsia due to disturbance of hypothalamic function. People with hyperthyroidism have their osmoreceptors reset and therefore feel thirstier than they should on the basis of their plasma osmolarity. It is thought that this may also be an important factor in causing polydipsia in cats.

(*continued overleaf*)

Table 12.1 (*continued*)

Disorder	Pathophysiology
Diabetes insipidus	Central diabetes insipidus is due to the absence of ADH, which results in impaired water and urea reabsorption from the distal collecting duct. This causes water loss as well as reduced osmolarity of the medullary interstitium due to reduced resorption of urea, which further reduces water reabsorption from the thin loop of Henle. Diabetes insipidus may be congenital or acquired (e.g. due to neoplasia, trauma or idiopathic). Nephrogenic diabetes insipidus is defined as lack of response to ADH. The most common cause is acquired impaired renal response to ADH as noted in Table 12.2. Congenital nephrogenic insipidus is very rare.
Hypercalcaemia	Hypercalcaemia impairs the action of ADH on the collecting duct, although the exact mechanism has not been identified. A protein, apical extracellular calcium-sensing receptor (CaSR), is believed to be involved. When luminal calcium increases, CaSR decreases ADH-induced permeability of the collecting duct. In addition, there may be down-regulation of the formation of water channels (aquaporin 2) in the collecting duct. The effect may be partial or total. Other mechanisms proposed include impaired Nacl transport in the loop of Henle and direct stimulation of the thirst centre. Hypercalcaemia will also decrease the glomerular filtration rate by causing vasoconstriction of afferent arterioles, which results initially in reversible azotaemia. Eventually, tubular function may become permanently impaired causing azotaemia due to nephrocalcinosis.
Hypokalaemia	Hypokalaemia results in mild to moderate impairment of urinary concentrating ability through ADH resistance. Aquaporin-2 is down-regulated, resulting in decreased permeability of the collecting duct to water.
Pyometra	Bacterial infection (*E. coli*) in pyometra causes decreased responsiveness to ADH, although urine dilution is still possible.

Table 12.1 *(continued)*

Disorder	Pathophysiology
Pyelonephritis	Pyelonephritis is an under-recognised cause of PU/PD. It causes PU/PD because interstitial inflammation in the kidney prevents the maintenance of the medullary concentrating gradient. The infective agent (particularly if it is *E. coli*) may also impair ADH function as occurs in patients with pyometra. Thus this is an example of a structural *and* functional mechanism causing impaired urine concentration. The severity of PU/PD can be marked. It is important to realise that patients with pyelonephritis can have PU/PD without becoming azotaemic, so they do not have renal failure *per se*. Impaired urine concentration is fully reversible when the infection resolves. It is also important to recognise that urinary tract infection limited to the lower urinary tract (i.e. an uncomplicated cystitis case) may result in pollakiuria and urgency but does not cause PU/PD.
Hypoadrenocorticism	Hyponatraemia due to any cause will impair urine concentration, although PU/PD may not be an overt clinical sign. The cause is related to decreased medullary osmolarity as a result of sodium loss. Low sodium also impairs the natural osmotic stimuli for ADH secretion (low serum osmolality) and so promotes dilute urine despite dehydration.
Diabetes mellitus	Primary polyuria in diabetes mellitus is due to the osmotic effect of glucose in the urine.
Chronic kidney disease	Both urine concentration and dilution are impaired in chronic kidney disease (CKD). As the number of functioning nephrons decreases, primary polyuria occurs partially due to osmotic diuresis as the remaining nephrons adapt and increase the fractional excretion of various solutes. Urea is probably the most important osmotic factor, and although the remaining nephrons cannot increase the fractional excretion of urea, the glomerular filtration rate (GFR) in the remaining nephrons does increase to a certain extent. There may also be distortion of medullary architecture, which disrupts the counter current mechanism. A relative insensitivity to ADH is also postulated.

- Decreased urea concentration in medullary interstitium
  - ADH deficiency/dysfunction (see point 4)
  - Liver disease?
- Hypercalcaemia, hypokalaemia, endotoxaemia and pyelonephritis can all impair the medullary concentration gradient through interference with normal tubular function

4. *Absence or interference with ADH function.* Some of the disorders that can produce PU/PD through this mechanism include the following:
   - Diabetes insipidus
   - Hyperadrenocorticism
   - Hypercalcaemia
   - Hypokalaemia
   - Pyometra
   - Pyelonephritis *especially if due to Escherichia coli*
5. *Osmotic diuresis.* Some of the disorders that can produce PU/PD through this mechanism include the following:
   - Glucosuria
     - Diabetes mellitus
     - Renal tubular defect.

Table 12.1 details the pathophysiological mechanisms causing PU/PD in various disorders.

Diagnostic approach to the patient with PU/PD or impaired urine concentration

1 Define the problem

The initial step in assessing the patient presenting with PU/PD is to ensure that true PU/PD is present, that is that increased drinking is not an appropriate physiological response. For example, animals with profuse watery diarrhoea will often drink more water than usual to maintain their hydration status. In addition, animals with gastritis will often drink large amounts of water but will vomit immediately and are not truly polydipsic. Exercise and high ambient temperatures may also induce an animal to drink more than usual – another appropriate physiological response. Those animals that drink excessively and subsequently urinate excessively (or vice versa) require investigation to determine the cause of their disordered water intake.

It is important to be aware that a polyuric animal may present for urinary incontinence, and the owner may not be aware or may not volunteer that the animal is drinking more than usual. However, owners may confuse pollakiuria with polyuria.

Confirmation of polydipsia

Polydipsia is usually defined in dogs as water intake that is twice maintenance requirements, that is approximately 100 mL/kg day. In cats, ingestion of greater than 50 mL/kg day is probably excessive and indicative of PU/PD. It may be necessary to measure the animal's water intake to ensure that it is polydipsic. However, particularly in the stressful hospital environment, a polydipsic animal may reduce its water intake for a period of time, and it is therefore desirable, if possible, to ask the owner to measure the intake at home.

Measurement at home, of course, may be very difficult or impossible if the owner has multiple animals and/or the pet drinks from uncontrolled sources such as pond, rain puddles or toilets. If the owner has noticed that the dog or cat is drinking substantially more often (especially cats), they can estimate roughly what the patient is drinking (e.g. 'I normally only have to fill the ice cream container once per day but now I have to fill it three times per day'), and if the urine (obtained by the owner or in the clinic) is not well concentrated, you can usually be fairly comfortable that the patient is polydipsic without having to accurately measure the water intake.

Related problems

There are other problems for which consideration of relevant pathophysiology and the diagnostic approach for PU/PD also applies.

If an animal is dehydrated or hypovolaemic, the appropriate renal response is to produce urine that is concentrated to at least a specific gravity (SG) of 1.030 (dogs) or 1.035 (cats). If a *dehydrated* animal has a urine SG less than 1.030, it has by definition *inadequate urine concentration,* and it must have some degree of renal dysfunction (primary structural renal dysfunction or extra-renal dysfunction).

If an *azotaemic* animal has a urine SG less than 1.030 (1.035 in cats), then the patient *must* have impaired urine concentrating ability, because if the azotaemia was *only* due to pre-renal factors *and* the patient had normal renal concentrating ability, the urine SG would be greater than 1.030 or 1.035.

Thus – the pathophysiological principles and diagnostic approach that follows in this chapter apply to three problems – which may or may not occur concurrently.

- Confirmed polydipsia
- Inappropriately dilute urine in a dehydrated patient
- Inappropriately dilute urine in an azotaemic patient.

Determine urine specific gravity

Having confirmed that an animal is truly polydipsic or polyuric, usually the initial and most important diagnostic step is to determine the urine SG – without this information, appropriate interpretation of other pathology results can be difficult. However, it is also important to consider the other clinical signs the patient may have, as this will have an important influence on consideration of realistic differentials. For example, if the patient is also polyphagic, the limited number of explanations allows the clinician to make a rational assessment of the likely diagnostic possibilities even before a urine sample is obtained.

- Urine with an *SG of less than 1.008* (1.006 in cats) has been actively diluted.
- Urine with an *SG of 1.008–1.012* has neither been diluted nor concentrated.
- Urine with an *SG of greater than 1.012* has been concentrated to some degree. However, whether the degree of concentration for the patient is appropriate must now be determined.

Normal animals may have a urine SG of any value depending on the physiological circumstances. It is therefore essential to always interpret urine SG *in relation to the hydration status of the patient.* Although urine with a SG greater than 1.012 has been concentrated to some extent, the degree of concentration may not be *appropriate* if there is any reason to suspect the patient has a diminished glomerular filtration rate – in other words, *if it is dehydrated or azotaemic or both.*

2 Define the system

Key question – structural or functional?

As stated previously, persistent polyuria is due to either primary polydipsia (effectively a behavioural abnormality) or a failure to concentrate urine appropriately. The latter may be the result of a *structural renal abnormality* (i.e. primary renal disease) or a *functional renal abnormality* (extra-renal disease).

A functional (extra-renal) abnormality occurs when urine concentration is impaired as a result of altered extra-renal factors that impinge on renal function, for example reduced renal medullary hypertonicity (as occurs with hyponatraemia) or diminished ADH function (as occurs with ADH deficiency and impaired ADH function secondary to other disorders such as hypercalcaemia, pyometra and hypokalaemia). In other words, the primary location of pathology does not lie within the kidney but elsewhere – the kidney is merely the 'messenger'.

If the urine is very dilute (hyposthenuria), there are a limited number of diagnostic possibilities (see Table 12.2), and differentiation of the possible causes is relatively simple. Structural renal disease (usually CKD), except pyelonephritis, can be ruled out because active dilution of urine into the hyposthenuric range requires the presence of normal numbers of nephrons.

If the urine SG is between 1.008 and 1.030, the first consideration is whether the urine is inappropriately dilute for the hydration status of the patient. If a patient is dehydrated and renal function is normal, the urine SG should be greater than 1.030 (dog) or 1.035 (cat). If it is not, then renal dysfunction *must* be present – this can be due to either a structural or a functional renal abnormality.

If the urine is concentrated, the patient was either *not* polyuric at the time of urine collection (which may occur in cases of primary polydipsia) or if it is definitely polyuric at the time of collection, then there must be an osmotic solute in the urine that is creating polyuria – the most common of these would be glucose.

Table 12.2 outlines the differential diagnoses for PU/PD or impaired urine concentration.

Having ascertained the urine concentration of the patient, the clinician can now concentrate on differentiating disorders that may be associated with each category.

3 Define the system/location

Hyposthenuria

Animals with persistent hyposthenuria *cannot* have CKD. Hyposthenuric urine has been actively diluted, a function that animals

Table 12.2 Differential diagnosis of *confirmed* polyuria/polydipsia or impaired urine concentration.

Urine concentration	Differential diagnosis	Useful tests
Hyposthenuria Urine SG <1.008	Psychogenic polydipsia	Water deprivation
	Diabetes insipidus*	Water deprivation/ADH response test
	Hypercalcaemia	Serum Ca^{2+} (total and ionised)
	Hyperadrenocorticism	Low dose dexamethasone suppression test and ACTH stimulation test
	Pyometra	Leukogram and abdominal diagnostic imaging
	Pyelonephritis	Urinalysis, urine culture and sensitivity
	Hepatic disease	ALT, ALP, bile acids and albumin
	Hypokalaemia	Serum K^+
	Hypoadrenocorticism (usually associated with isosthenuria or hypersthenuria but occasionally can cause hyposthenuria)	Leukogram, serum Na^{2+}, Na^+:K^+ ratio, basal cortisol and ACTH stimulation test
Lack of appropriate concentration Urine SG 1.008–1.030	Chronic kidney disease (CKD)	Urea, creatinine and PO^{-4}, iohexol
	Hypercalcaemia	Serum Ca^{2+} (total and ionised)
	Hyperadrenocorticism	Low dose dexamethasone suppression test and ACTH stimulation test
	Hepatic disease	ALT, ALP and bile acids
	Diabetes mellitus	Blood and urine glucose
	Pyometra	Leukogram and abdominal diagnostic imaging

(*continued overleaf*)

Table 12.2 (*continued*)

Urine concentration	Differential diagnosis	Useful tests
	Pyelonephritis	Urinalysis, urine culture and sensitivity
	Hyponatraemia	Serum Na^{2+}, Na^+:K^+ ratio, resting cortisol and ACTH stimulation test
	Hypokalaemia	Serum K^+
Concentrated Urine SG >1.030	Diabetes mellitus	Urine and blood glucose
	Renal glucosuria	Urine and blood glucose

Further Comments Related to Table 12.2

- Animals with partial central diabetes insipidus (low but not total lack of ADH) can have isosthenuric urine *if* they are dehydrated.
- Animals with partial diabetes insipidus (central or nephrogenic) may on occasions have both hyposthenuria and isosthenuria.
- Other disorders that may be associated with polyuria/polydipsia and SG values ranging from hyposthenuric to concentrated include *hyperthyroidism, polycythaemia* and *pheocromocytoma, multiple myeloma and primary hypoparathyroidism.*
- Polyuria will occur in the diuretic phase of acute renal failure and post urinary tract obstruction.

with CKD cannot perform. Therefore, by definition, all patients with PU/PD and hyposthenuria have a functional renal abnormality. As noted in Table 12.1, pyelonephritis poses a conceptual challenge as there are structural changes in the kidney (inflammation), but the mechanism for PU/PD involves alteration of the interstitial concentration gradient (as well as ADH dysfunction), *not* brought about by an absolute *reduction in the number* of nephrons as in CKD but by impaired *function* of the otherwise adequate number of nephrons present.

Persistent hyposthenuria is a consistent feature of central diabetes insipidus and may also be present in patients with primary polydipsia. Note, however, that a patient with partial central diabetes insipidus may present with urine with a SG greater than 1.008.

Hyperadrenocorticism, liver disease, pyometra, hyperthyroidism, hyponatraemia, pyelonephritis and hypercalcaemia may all be associated with hyposthenuria but, as Table 12.2 illustrates, can also be associated with urine SG in the range 1.008–1.030.

Dogs with internal haemorrhage, for example due to splenic haemangiosarcoma, can present with profound PU/PD and hyposthenuria. This is paradoxical because haemorrhage is a potent stimulus for ADH release, as ADH at high doses has a vasopressor function (hence its other name, vasopressin). This should cause increased urine concentration and hemodilution due to water retention. The observed polyuria and hyposthenuria is a compensatory measure stimulated by the initial haemodilution (excretion of excess water) compounded by the stimulation of the thirst mechanism by hypovolaemia due to profound blood loss.

When should a water deprivation test be performed?

A water deprivation test should *not* be the first procedure performed once hyposthenuria is confirmed. Animals with hepatic disease, hypercalcaemia, hyperadrenocorticism, hyperthyroidism, hyponatraemia and pyometra may or may not be able to concentrate urine to a certain extent and a water deprivation test will be of little discriminatory value. Note that azotaemia is an *absolute* contraindication to performing a water deprivation test – if the patient is azotaemic, it has in essence failed the test.

In addition, water deprivation and delay in diagnosis may be detrimental, particularly to animals with hypercalcaemia (we can probably assume that an animal with pyometra will have sufficient other clinical signs to ensure that a diagnosis is made relatively easily). Therefore, the first step should be directed at determining whether hepatic disease, hyperadrenocorticism, pyometra, hyperthyroidism, pyelonephritis or hypercalcaemia exists.

A diagnosis of PU/PD associated with hepatic disease (most often, hepatic encephalopathy), hypercalcaemia, hyperthyroidism, hypoadrenocorticism, pyelonephritis or pyometra can be made relatively easily based on the history, physical examination and selected tests.

Thus, the time to consider a water deprivation test is when dealing with a PU/PD patient with hyposthenuria who has continued to drink excessively despite a period of hospitalisation and where there are no indications of the potential for the aforementioned extra-renal disorders resulting in ADH insensitivity. In other words, attempting to differentiate ADH deficiency from a patient with primary polydipsia who continues to drink excessively despite a period of altered environment (see further discussion in the following sections).

4 Define the lesion

Differentiating causes of hyposthenuria

Hepatic disease

Hepatic disease is usually associated with other clinical signs in addition to PU/PD and can be investigated by measurement of serum enzymes and bile acids if serum enzymology is only slightly abnormal. However, note that up to 25% of patients with confirmed hepatobiliary disease may have bile acids values less than 25 μm/L.

Hypercalcaemia

Hypercalcaemia can be diagnosed by a serum calcium level – preferably ionised as well as total. It is usually associated with systemic signs such as inappetence and/or gastrointestinal signs, although patients with primary hypoparathyroidism can appear surprisingly well.

Pyometra

Patients with pyometra will have other clinical signs as well as PU/PD and should not pose a diagnostic dilemma.

Pyelonephritis

Pyelonephritis is an under-recognised cause of PU/PD. Urinalysis may have clues that a urinary tract infection is present but they can be subtle, and the absence, for example, of haematuria or proteinuria does not necessarily rule the diagnosis out. Urine culture and susceptibility are strongly recommended in any patient with PU/PD if an explanation has not been found from appropriate blood tests.

Hyperthyroidism

Hyperthyroidism is primarily of consideration in cats and will usually be associated with other clinical signs and increased serum T4 values.

Hyperadrenocorticism

The diagnosis of hyperadrenocorticism may prove more problematical, as animals may not have any other clinical signs (although some will have characteristic signs such as alopecia, thin skin, pot belly and hepatomegaly).

Although a low dose dexamethasone suppression test is necessary to definitively diagnose or exclude hyperadrenocorticism, the vast majority of animals with the disorder will have increased ALP and/or cholesterol and/or stress leukogram. Thus, a polydipsic animal that has *no* other clinical signs and *no* changes in these haematological or biochemical parameters is unlikely to have hyperadrenocorticism, although the diagnosis cannot be completely excluded without provocative adrenal testing.

Dogs with hyperadrenocorticism are usually systemically well (i.e. they eat well and are fairly bright and alert). If the dog is systemically unwell, then non-adrenal illness should be suspected (even if there is also concurrent hyperadrenocorticism).

The low dose dexamethasone suppression test and ACTH stimulation test can be abnormal in systemically unwell animals with non-adrenal disease, and hence it is very important to interpret these tests in light of the dog's overall well-being. If there is concurrent illness but you still suspect that hyperadrenocorticism may be present, delay provocative testing of the adrenal gland until the concurrent disease has been resolved and the dog appears systemically well.

What if all the tests are normal?

If an animal with PU/PD, hyposthenuria and no other clinical signs has a normal white blood cell count, serum calcium, serum ALP and ALT, serum T4, fasting and postprandial bile acids, albumin and serum cholesterol and a negative urine culture, then closed pyometra, hypercalcaemia, hyperthyroidism, pyelonephritis and probably hepatic disease can be eliminated from the differential diagnosis (hepatic encephalopathy can definitely be eliminated, but bile acids are less sensitive to other types of liver pathology and can be normal even in advanced disease). Hyperadrenocorticism is unlikely but is theoretically possible and should be investigated by a low dose dexamethasone suppression test or ACTH stimulation test.

Diabetes insipidus vs. primary polydipsia

The clinician can now concentrate on differentiating diabetes insipidus from primary polydipsia due to behavioural causes – what has sometimes been described as psychogenic polydipsia. Animals with primary polydipsia will often alter their water intake in a different environment, and a pragmatic approach before embarking on specific testing can be to hospitalise the patient and measure water intake. If water intake falls to normal, then the diagnosis of primary polydipisa is made. If it does not, then assuming all other causes of primary polydipsia and primary polyuria have been excluded, diabetes insipidus and primary polydipsia may be differentiated by a water deprivation test.

It is important to recognise that the end point of a water deprivation test must be detectable dehydration, which may take many hours in an animal with normal urine-concentrating capacity. In contrast, the animal with diabetes insipidus has no capacity to concentrate urine in the face of water deprivation and hence can become dehydrated extremely quickly (within hours). Close monitoring of body weight, PCV, plasma protein and blood urea is essential to prevent catastrophic hypernatraemia occurring. It is not acceptable, for example, to deprive the animal of water overnight and see what its urine SG is in the morning – the chances are you'll have a moribund patient with a brain as dry as a crisp if it does have diabetes insipidus.

Animals with primary polydipsia will usually be able to concentrate urine appropriately, although occasionally, medullary washout secondary to profound polyuria may impair concentration. A partial water deprivation test with or without salt administration may be necessary in some cases. If you are considering a water deprivation test to rule out primary polydipsia, it is often a good idea to get the owner to collect multiple urine samples from different times of the day. Often, these dogs will only have low urine SGs some of the time (because they can concentrate their urine if they are not drinking excessively). For example, after a long walk is a good time to get a concentrated sample. Then you have no need to do a water deprivation test.

ADH response test

If the patient has been water deprived for sufficient time to induce dehydration, their urine SG remains in the hyposthenuric range and hyperadrenocorticism, hypercalcaemia, hepatic disease, hyperthyroidism, pyelonephritis and pyometra have been ruled out by appropriate testing, central diabetes insipidus is the most probable diagnosis and response to ADH should be assessed.

A positive response to ADH (2.5–5.0 units Pitressin tannate im or 0.5 U/kg aqueous ADH im) confirms central diabetes insipidus. If pitressin tannate is unavailable, desmopressin acetate (Minirin) drops can be instilled in the eye. A negative response suggests a diagnosis of nephrogenic diabetes insipidus (a very rare and controversial diagnosis).

Pragmatically, it is often safer and more expedient to perform a desmopressin response test without a prior water deprivation test in a dog where there is a very high index of suspicion of diabetes insipidus.

Urine SG greater than 1.008

A urine SG from 1.008 to 1.035 is only evidence of a urine-concentrating defect if the patient is definitely PU/PD and/or dehydrated and/or azotaemic.

As Table 12.2 illustrates, the differential diagnoses for the animal with inappropriately dilute urine when the urine concentration is 1.008–1.035 include renal disease, hyperadrenocorticism, diabetes mellitus, hypercalcaemia, pyometra, hyperthyroidism, hypokalaemia, hypoadrenocorticism, pyelonephritis and hepatic disease (or very occasionally, consider diabetes insipidus if the patient is dehydrated).

Diagnostic approach

As discussed in the previous section, hepatic disease, pyometra, hypercalcaemia, hyperthyroidism, hypoadrencorticism, pyelonephritis and hyperadrenocorticism can be excluded relatively easily from the list of differential diagnoses by routine tests.

Diabetes mellitus is also easily investigated using urine and/or blood glucose levels (note that cats may have substantial hyperglycaemia associated with stress and other disease, and animals with proximal renal tubular defects may have glucosuria without hyperglycaemia). Hypokalaemia may be investigated by measuring serum potassium concentrations.

CKD, however, can pose a diagnostic challenge. Animals with impaired urine concentration due to CKD may or may not be azotaemic depending on the percentage of nephron loss – loss of 67% of nephron function results in impaired concentration ability, and loss of 75% results in azotaemia.

Animals with pyelonephritis can be identified based on urinalysis and urine culture. Renal imaging may also provide clues. These patients do not necessarily have CKD, and their impaired ability to concentrate their urine is reversible once the infection has resolved.

Water deprivation test useful?

Although it is often assumed that a water deprivation test is useful in diagnosing compensated (non-azotaemic) renal disease, it should be remembered that the animal with compensated CKD may become seriously azotaemic if water is deprived and dehydration ensues. As previously mentioned, disorders such as hyperadrenocorticism may also impair the animal's ability to concentrate urine in the face of dehydration, and hence the test may not be particularly discriminatory. It is preferable to rule out other possible disorders with appropriate tests as outlined in Table 12.2. If these tests are all normal and there are no other clinical signs, CKD is the probable diagnosis. Confirmation requires more sophisticated tests to measure glomerular filtration rate, such as endogenous or exogenous creatinine clearance (not usually feasible in practice).

It is important to recognise that hypercalcaemia and hypoadrenocorticism (or hyponatraemia due to other causes) as well as CKD may be associated with impaired urine concentration and azotaemia even if the patient is not dehydrated (see Table 12.3).

Concentrated urine

The most common diagnosis in this category is diabetes mellitus.

Note that polyuria in diabetes mellitus is due to the osmotic effect of glucose in the renal tubules, which decreases water reabsorption from, for example, the thin loop of Henle. Urine concentrating ability *itself*, however, is not impaired, as the extra water excreted is accompanied by a solute (glucose) and there is no disturbance to medullary hypertonicity.

Table 12.3 Summary of mechanisms for azotaemia and impaired urine concentration.

Disorder	Reason for decreased glomerular filtration rate (GFR) resulting in azotaemia	Reason for impaired urine concentration
Structural renal disease	Decreased number of functional nephrons	Decreased number of functional nephrons
Hypercalcaemia	Constricted afferent arteriole +/− decreased renal perfusion if patient dehydrated	ADH dysfunction
Hyponatraemia	Hypovolaemia due to reduced blood volume associated with decrease serum sodium +/− decreased renal perfusion if patient dehydrated	Decreased medullary hypertonicity Impaired ADH release in dehydration
Dehydrated patient with normal renal function	Decreased renal perfusion	Urine concentration not impaired
Dehydrated patient with polyuric disorder	Decreased renal perfusion	ADH dysfunction or osmotic diuresis or reduced medullary hypertonicity
Glomerular disease	Decreased rate of flow through glomerulus	Not impaired until tubular pathology develops

Renal glucosuria vs. diabetes mellitus

Renal tubular defects causing glucosuria should also be considered and differentiated from diabetes mellitus by measuring blood glucose.

Cats with stress-related hyperglycaemia may also have glucosuria that could conceivably be of sufficient magnitude to cause polyuria. Diagnosis of the underlying disorder can present a challenge in these patients. However, measurement of serum fructosamine levels is useful in differentiating most cases of stress hyperglycaemia from true diabetes mellitus.

Animals with hyperadrenocorticism, hypercalcaemia and hypoadrenocorticism may not be consistently polyuric and, therefore, may have concentrated urine at certain times.

In conclusion

Assessment of the patient with PU/PD can be relatively simple and straightforward for common disorders but more complex in other cases. Although referring to a list of differential diagnoses such as Table 12.2 can be helpful in assessing PU/PD cases, an understanding of the pathophysiological basis for impaired urine concentration assists enormously in the rational interpretation of appropriate diagnostic tests so that the diagnosis can be reached expediently and safely.

CHAPTER 13
Gait abnormalities

Holger A. Volk & Elvin R. Kulendra
The Royal Veterinary College, Department of Clinical Science and Services, London, UK

Introduction

Differentiating between causes of gait abnormalities in practice can be challenging. However, by initially defining the problem and the system involved, a list of further appropriate diagnostic tests can be performed. Despite the recent advances in diagnostic imaging, the neurological and orthopaedic examinations remain the foundation of localising the lesion. The majority of cats and dogs that present with a thoracic or pelvic limb lameness will have an underlying orthopaedic condition, but it is important to recognise that neurological disorders can present with similar clinical signs. Neurological disorders will more commonly present as decreased voluntary movement (paresis) or lack of voluntary movement (plegia).

Once the location of the lesion has been defined, a list of differential diagnoses can be formulated based on signalment, onset, clinical course and clinical features such as pain and asymmetry of clinical signs. Each individual case has its own challenges, and any purely rule-based system is likely to result in mistakes. However, this chapter proposes an approach to gait abnormalities that will help the reader define the problem, system, location and lesion to help identify the most appropriate diagnostic route.

Clinical Reasoning in Small Animal Practice, First Edition.
Jill E. Maddison, Holger A. Volk and David B. Church.

Differentiating musculoskeletal from neurological gait abnormalities

1 Define the problem

The first step when an animal presents with gait abnormalities should be to define the problem. A gait abnormality is any change in the normal gait pattern for that animal or deviation from the typical gait of the same species. Defining the problem for an animal with a gait abnormality primarily involves information given by the owner and observation by the clinician. Clarifying whether the patient is lame on one or more legs, if there is a shifting lameness, change in stride length, if the gait is stilted, if the patient is stiff (and if so where and when), if leg movement is abnormal (e.g. bunny hopping), if the animal appears weak, if they are ataxic and so on are all important in progressing understanding of the abnormality present and the likely differential diagnoses. Lameness can be defined as decreased weight bearing of the affected limb or an altered gait, and animals may shift their weight on to their other limbs to compensate.

2 Define the system

The majority of patients who present with gait abnormalities will have an underlying orthopaedic or neurological disorder. The problem may be due to an underlying structural or functional disease process. Both structural and functional disorders can lead to weakness, difficulty rising, collapse and gait alterations. Weakness can be defined as reduced muscle strength, which can manifest as difficulty rising and lack of movement. This is discussed in more detail in Chapter 6.

A primary structural problem can involve the musculoskeletal system or nervous system (neuromuscular/peripheral nervous system [PNS] or central nervous system [CNS]). A functional abnormality can be caused by derangements of the cardiovascular, respiratory or metabolic systems that have a secondary effect on the nervous or musculoskeletal system, for example hypoglycaemia secondary to an insulinoma. Typically, functional abnormalities that result in alteration of the gait will have concurrent clinical signs that may be related to other body systems. For example, it would not be unusual for a dog with an insulinoma to present with seizures as well as weakness.

Those patients who have structural abnormalities in multiple locations, for example, musculoskeletal as well as the nervous system, can prove to be a challenge, as it can be difficult to identify which is the most clinically significant problem. However, a thorough scrutiny of the history and physical examination may give the clinician clues.

Abnormalities of any of the following systems can results in clinical signs of weakness (Chapter 6), collapse (Chapter 7) or gait abnormalities.

- Primary structural
  - Musculoskeletal – muscles, bones, ligaments, tendons and joints
  - Nervous – CNS and neuromuscular system
- Secondary functional
  - Cardiovascular – heart, vascular structures and blood
  - Metabolic – electrolytes, for example potassium/sodium and glucose
  - Respiratory – upper or lower airways, pleural space and thoracic wall.

The presence of concurrent clinical signs, history and laboratory work will generally allow the clinician to prioritise the body systems in order of clinical significance. The diagnostic approach to weakness and collapse is discussed elsewhere (Chapters 6 and 7), and this chapter concentrates on other gait abnormalities, primarily lameness.

The majority of patients who present with gait abnormalities will have abnormalities that primarily and structurally affect either the musculoskeletal or the nervous systems. As a result, lesion localisation will concentrate on lesions affecting the musculoskeletal and neurological systems. Unlike the cardiovascular, metabolic and respiratory body systems, there is no simple laboratory or diagnostic test that can be performed to differentiate between the nervous and musculoskeletal body systems. The differentiation between the two systems is based on the clinician's physical examination. Figure 13.1 can be used as an aid to help identify whether the clinical signs identified are to be more likely associated with musculoskeletal (orthopaedic) or nervous system (neurological) disease.

Most animals with neurological disorders will present with paresis, while those with orthopaedic disorders will present with lameness.

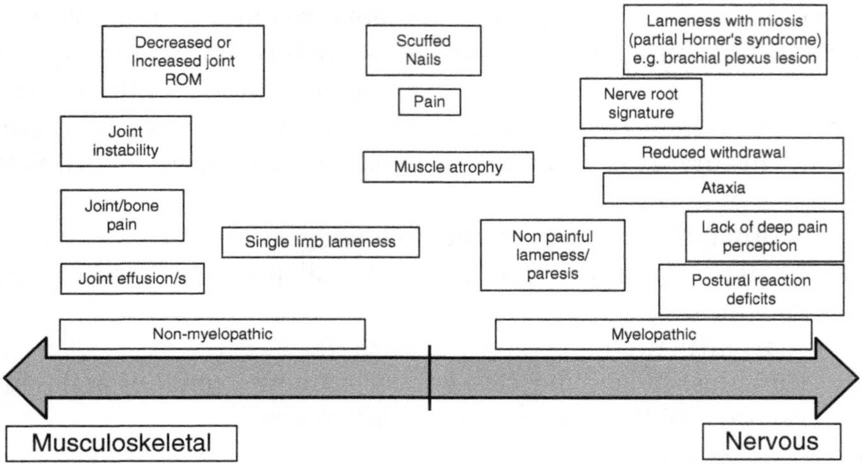

Figure 13.1 Clinical deficits to help differentiate between musculoskletal and nervous system disorders (ROM=range of movement).

It can be challenging to differentiate lameness (inability to move) and paresis (inability to create movement). It is not uncommon for patients with bilateral orthopaedic disease, for example bilateral cruciate disease, to present in a similar manner to those with neurological disorders. However, the most challenging cases involve those patients where both orthopaedic and neurological disorders coexist.

3 Define the location

The location of the problem can be identified by a systematic and thorough orthopaedic and neurological examination. Following the examination, the clinician will hopefully be able to localise the lesion. If the orthopaedic system is involved, structures affected include the long bones, joints, muscles, tendons or ligamentous structures. However, if the lesion involves the neurological system, the lesion may affect the CNS and PNS. Most parts of the nervous system (brain, spinal cord or neuromuscular system) can be associated with gait abnormalities (also see Chapter 6). CNS dysfunction can involve the forebrain ('initiation of movement'), cerebellum ('fine-tuning of movement') or brainstem ('motor coordination and long fibre tracts passing to the target muscles'). Lesions affecting these brain structures can be usually easily differentiated from orthopaedic gait abnormalities, as they are accompanied by other brain-specific deficits such as behaviour and mentation changes, cranial nerve deficits and/or vestibular deficits (Chapter 7). Deficits of the neuromuscular system or the spinal cord, however, can be more difficult to differentiate from orthopaedic problems. How to localise and characterise the lesion in these compartments will be discussed in the following section.

History

Before an orthopaedic or neurological examination, it is important to obtain a thorough history. A complete history can provide vital information relevant to the underlying aetiology of the lameness and the appropriate next diagnostic step(s). A general history regarding the animal's overall systemic health should be obtained before focusing on more specific questions regarding the gait. A general outline to obtain a more specific history for gait abnormalities is listed as follows:

- Signalment
- Which leg(s) is (are) affected?
- What is the clinical onset and chronological progression of the gait abnormality?
- Is it worse after exercise/after rising from recumbency?
- Progression of the gait abnormality – is it deteriorating, stable or improving?
- Response to medication/rest?
- Any history of lameness in other limbs?
- Any changes in behaviour or mentation?
- Any history of back pain?
- Has there been a history of pyrexia?
- Has there been any weight loss?

Once a history has been obtained, a general examination should be performed to identify any other concurrent conditions that may be significant. This is especially important after trauma, as it helps to identify life-threatening injuries that should be addressed before treatment of the animal's orthopaedic or neurological injuries.

Orthopaedic examination

The orthopaedic examination is the key to identify the location of the lesion, and therefore the examination is discussed in detail in this chapter. It can be divided into three parts: distant examination, gait analysis and palpation/manipulation. The first two parts of the examination may be performed without sedation, but in extremely painful or aggressive patients, the final part may need to be performed under general anaesthesia or sedation.

Distant examination

Examination should begin with distant observation of the animal standing or sitting. The examiner should take time to observe for evidence of muscle atrophy. This is most evident over the proximal thigh muscles in the pelvic limbs and over the spine of the scapula in the thoracic limbs. The amount of weight distributed through the individual thoracic and pelvic limbs should be noted. Is weight distribution symmetrical? When the animal is standing straight, the examiner should assess for any evidence of limb malalignment, for example, carpal varus/valgus. Observing the animal rising to standing from lying down may demonstrate that it favours one particular limb when rising. It may be possible to diagnose the problem solely from distant observation; for example, contracture of the infraspinatus has a characteristic posture of elbow abduction and external rotation of the lower limb.

Gait analysis

Following distant examination, the animal should be observed walking and trotting. In selected cases, walking the animal up and down the stairs can also help identify lameness. Walking up the steps will exacerbate pelvic limb lameness, whereas walking down steps will exacerbate any thoracic limb lameness. A long well-lit corridor is beneficial, but an outdoor private road or car park can also be used. Some animals may struggle or panic on the slippery floors inside the hospital, and the outside road may be more appropriate for the examination of these animals. Certain lameness can also be exacerbated when the animal is walked on hard surfaces and become easily identifiable from the transition from grass to concrete, for example, digital corns.

The animal should be initially walked on a lead. The lead should have enough slack in it so that a head nod is not masked. The animal is walked slowly up and down the corridor. When the animal is turned, it is important that the animal is kept on the inside of the dog walker so that the gait can be assessed during this phase of the examination. The speed is gradually increased to a trot. If the lameness is only present during running, this part of the examination is best accomplished in a confined secure area. If this is not possible, the authors would recommend that the owner takes a video of the lameness. For cats, observation should be performed in the examination room.

When the animal is being walked or trotted, the presence of a head nod in the thoracic limb is consistent with a thoracic limb lameness. When the lame leg hits the ground, the head will rise, and when the sound leg hits the ground, the leg will sink ('SSS: sink on sound side'). Stride length should also be assessed, as animals with bilateral lameness will have shortened stride lengths present. Nails should be assessed for any evidence of scuffing, and the animal should also be assessed for evidence of ataxia (incoordination). The lameness can be graded from a scale of 0–10, with 0 representing a sound animal, and 10 representing a non-weight-bearing lameness. Lameness grading is most useful as a subjective measure of lameness during follow-up examinations when performed by the same observer. Certain conditions have a characteristic gait, for example gracilis contracture. Dogs with gracilis contracture internally rotate the leg during stifle extension and have a shortened stride length. The result is a characteristic 'flicking' of the distal limb.

Physical examination

An orthopaedic examination is always performed following a thorough general physical examination. By this point in the assessment, the distant examination and gait analysis would hopefully have allowed localisation of the lameness to a particular limb. The orthopaedic examination will subsequently allow the source of the *lameness to be localised to the bone, joint(s), muscle, tendon or ligaments* that are involved. Ideally, the patient should be examined before sedation or general anaesthesia, the animal's temperament permitting.

The examination should be performed in a methodical manner to ensure that a cause of the lameness is not over looked. The brain has a natural bias to focus on the most severely affected leg, and one can easily overlook the other legs being affected, which can then misguide your clinical decision-making. The affected leg should be examined last to prevent upsetting the patient before a complete examination can be performed. The animal is palpated for signs of asymmetry in muscle mass in the thoracic and pelvic limbs. The authors routinely palpate the muscles of the proximal thigh muscles in the pelvic limb and the supraspinatus and infraspinatus in the thoracic limbs to assess muscle atrophy. The supraspinatus is cranial to the spine of the scapula and the infraspinatus caudal to it.

Pressure is then placed on the palmar/plantar aspect of the carpus or tarsus while the animal is standing to assess the degree of weight bearing of each limb. It is important to make sure that the dog is standing square at this point. The neck is flexed and extended dorsally, ventrally and laterally. Palpation of the cervical, thoracic and lumbar spine is performed. Animals with lumbosacral pain often react when the tail is elevated dorsally. If abnormalities are detected, a full neurological examination is warranted.

Small dogs are most easily examined on the table-top, but larger dogs are often examined on the floor. The patient is examined in lateral recumbency, but if the animal does not tolerate this, it can be performed with the animal standing. All four limbs are examined starting from the toes and moving proximally. If the lesion is in the paw, starting the examination proximally and moving distally will help with cooperation of the patient. Generally, each joint should be examined for any evidence of swelling, restriction in range of movement, pain, signs of instability and crepitus. The long bones should be palpated for signs of pain, for example, neoplasia or panosteitis. Lymph nodes should also be assessed for any signs of enlargement. The prescapular (superficial cervical) and axillary lymph nodes are assessed in the thoracic limbs and the popliteal and inguinal lymph nodes in the pelvic limbs.

Thoracic limbs

Each toe is individually examined as well as the inderdigital space. Pressure is applied over the digital pads individually, and the pads are checked for signs of trauma. This is a common site for corns. The individual digits and phalangeal joints are palpated. Moving proximally, the metacarpophalangeal joints are examined, and pressure is applied over the palmar aspect of the joint over the sesamoid bones to assess for pain (e.g. pain may be associated with fragmentation of sesamoid bones II and VII in Rottweilers). The metacarpal bones are carefully palpated to the level of the carpus. Effusion of the carpus will be most prominent on the dorsal aspect of the joint at the level of the antebrachiocarpal joint. The joint should be assessed for any evidence of pain on flexion/extension or for signs of instability following valgus/varus/palmar/dorsal stresses applied to the joint.

Pressure is applied to the antebrachium moving distally to proximally. Pain on palpation over the antebrachium should lead the clinician to review the structures that may be involved (e.g. tenosynovitis of the abductor pollicis longus often presents with swelling and pain over the medial aspect of the distal radius). The elbow is fully flexed and extended, and firm pressure is applied over the medial and lateral aspect of the humeral epicondyles.

An elbow effusion is most noticeable on the lateral aspect of the joint between the lateral epicondyle and the olecranon. Comparison of the contralateral side can be useful for subtle joint effusions.

Normal range of movement in the elbow is approximately 35° in flexion and 165° in extension. When the elbow is flexed, the antebrachium can be pronated and supinated concurrently. Certain conditions such as medial compartment disease of the elbow may be more painful on flexion and pronation of the antebrachium at the same time. Care must be taken to avoid manipulation of the carpus at the same time. When the elbow and carpus are maintained at 90° and the antebrachium is pronated and supinated, the integrity of the collateral ligaments can be assessed (Campbell's test). The Campbell's test can be useful for assessing the stability of the elbow joint following closed reduction of an elbow luxation.

Pressure is applied to the humerus working proximally towards the shoulder. The radial nerve runs in a caudoproximal to craniodistal direction in the distal third of the humerus. Care is taken to ensure that pressure is applied directly to the bone. During palpation, the contour of the bone should be assessed for any irregularities. The large triceps muscle mass is caudal to the humerus and inserts on the olecranon. The triceps tendon can be easily palpated when the elbow is in extension. The biceps is found cranial to the humerus.

The shoulder joint lies just distal to the acromion but is relatively deep, and as such, a joint effusion can be difficult to appreciate.

Pathology of the biceps tendon is exacerbated with the shoulder in full flexion, whilst the elbow is maintained in extension. Pressure is then exerted over the biceps as it runs through the intertubercular groove; the groove is medial to the greater tubercle of the humerus. Shoulder instability may be apparent with the measurement of the shoulder abduction angle. A normal dog will have approximately 30° of shoulder abduction. Dogs with brachial plexus tumours may be painful on deep palpation of the axillary region.

Pelvic limbs

The authors start with the dog standing and assesses the muscle mass of the proximal thigh muscles on the left and right sides. This is often a good indicator of lameness if there is muscle atrophy over one side. Dogs with bilateral disease will have bilateral muscle atrophy. With the animal still standing, the greater trochanter, ischiatic tuberosity and the cranial aspect of the dorsal iliac spine are located. A triangular shape should be formed between the three points. However, in cases where there is craniodorsal coxofemoral luxation, the greater trochanter becomes displaced dorsally and the three points will form a straight line. The size and shape of the triangle that is formed should be symmetrical between the left and the right side (pelvic fractures will often result in pelvic asymmetry).

If the patient will tolerate it, the animal is placed in lateral recumbency and the examination starts distally as described for the thoracic limbs. At the level of the hock, the joint should be flexed and extended. The range of movement in the normal tarsocrural joint is 40° in flexion and 165° in extension in the dog. The cat has more flexion (22°) compared to the dog. Flexion and extension of the hock will result in passive flexion and extension of the stifle joint; the exception to this would be when there is disruption to the Achilles tendon. In this scenario, the hock will be able to be extended and flexed independently of the stifle. When the hock is kept in extension, the Achilles tendon is placed under less tension, and it is easier to appreciate any abnormalities in the tendon.

Effusion of the hock can be palpated medially and laterally, dorsal and plantar to the malleolus. When the hock is examined for instability, it is important that the joint is stressed medial to lateral, dorsal to plantar and for rotational instability. Cats inherently will have more laxity in the tarsus than dogs, and comparison with the contralateral limb can be useful in the detection of subtle abnormalities. Instability at the tarsocrural joint can be identified by stabilising the medial and lateral malleolus with one hand and grasping the base of the metatarsus with the other. Intertarsal instability can be identified by grasping the calcaneus with one hand and the base of the metatarsus with the other (e.g. calcaneoquartal instability seen in Shetland sheepdogs secondary to degeneration of the plantar tarsal ligament).

The cranial and medial aspects of the tibia are covered by a thin layer of soft tissues. Both the lateral malleolus of the fibula and the medial malleolus of the tibia can be palplated distally. Moving proximally, the tibial tuberosity (insertion of the patellar ligament) can be palpated. The patellar ligament should be easily palpable as a distinct band that runs between the tibial tuberosity and the patella. In cases where there is a stifle effusion, the margins of the patellar ligament become less distinct. The fibula head lies just distal to the lateral femoral condyle. The lateral fabella (sesamoid bone within the lateral belly of the gastrocnemius tendon) lies just proximal to the fibula head. The normal stifle joint has a range of motion of approximately 120°, 40° in flexion and 160° in extension. Cranial drawer and tibial thrust are specific tests that are used to assess the integrity of the cranial cruciate ligament. Cranial drawer is performed by stabilising the femur with one hand and the proximal tibia with the other. The thumbs and index finger should form a square. The hand stabilising the femur should have the thumb over the lateral fabella and the index finger over the patella. The tibia should be stabilised with the index finger over the tibial tuberosity and the thumb over the fibula head. The femur should be maintained in a fixed position while the tibia is moved in a cranial direction. The test should be performed in flexion and extension, as partial ruptures of the cranial cruciate ligament may only be detectable in flexion. Full extension of the stifle may result in a false negative result, as the collateral ligaments remain taut in extension preventing cranial translation of the tibia.

Tibial thrust is an alternative to cranial drawer to assess the integrity of the cruciate ligament. This test may be easier to perform in the conscious animal and in large/giant breed dogs. The test is performed by stabilising the cranial aspect of the distal femur with one hand and placing the index finger over the tibial tuberosity.

The other hand grasps the metatarsus. The stifle is maintained at a fixed angle and the hock is flexed. Cruciate deficient stifles will result in cranial translation of the tibial tuberosity. The manoeuvre should be performed at various angles of flexion and extension.

To assess for patellar luxation, the stifle is best maintained in extension, and pressure is applied to the patella medially and laterally. The author also assesses the severity of the patellar luxation when the dog is weight bearing. If the patella is difficult to identify, the tibial tuberosity is identified first, and the patellar ligament is palpated to the level of the patella. Pressure can be applied directly over the patella, and this can be useful in identifying dogs that have retropatellar pain. The femur can be difficult to palpate due to the large amount of soft tissue musculature present, the exception being the femoral condyles and the greater trochanter.

The hip is a ball and socket joint that allows the joint to move in three dimensions. Extension and flexion of the hip are initially performed, but more specific tests can be performed when the dog is under general anaesthesia or deeply sedated. The Ortolani and Bardens tests are commonly used to assess for hip instability in dogs that have hip dysplasia. The Ortolani test involves placing the dog in dorsal recumbency, and the femurs are placed perpendicular to the spine. The stifle joint is stabilised, and pressure is applied towards the spine/table to subluxate the hips dorsally. The femur is slowly abducted until a palpable 'clunk' is appreciated. This corresponds to reduction of the femoral head back into the acetabulum; this is known as the 'angle of reduction'. The femur is then adducted until the hip reluxates; this is known as the 'angle of luxation'. Bardens test involves holding the medial stifle and distal femur and placing the thumb of the other hand on the greater trochanter. Lateral displacement is applied to the femur to appreciate the amount of laxity that is present. Displacement of greater than 1–2 cm is probably abnormal.

Lastly, a rectal examination to assess the prostate in male dogs and the sublumbar lymph nodes should be performed. Male dogs with prostatic disease can present with a pelvic limb lameness or difficulty rising. Intrapelvic masses may also be identified following rectal examination as a cause of pelvic limb lameness. Based on physical examination findings, Figure 13.3 can be used as a guide to identify the appropriate diagnostic step(s) in the investigation.

Neurological examination

The neurological examination relies on patient's compliance as does the orthopaedic examination. Try to perform the neurological examination in a way that the animal feels comfortable. Otherwise, especially proprioceptive tests can result in false positives. General observations (mentation, posture and gait) should be completed first, and assessments with the potential to cause pain (palpation and nociception) should be left until last. Ideally, a complete neurological examination is performed, but in some patients, this may not be possible. The order of the examination can be arranged so that tests that are more clinically relevant to the presenting complaint can be evaluated earlier (and hopefully before patient compliance is lost). In cases where one is uncertain about the neurological localisation, repeating the neurological examination may increase the likelihood of recognising subtle abnormalities. It may also reveal trends in the progression of clinical signs.

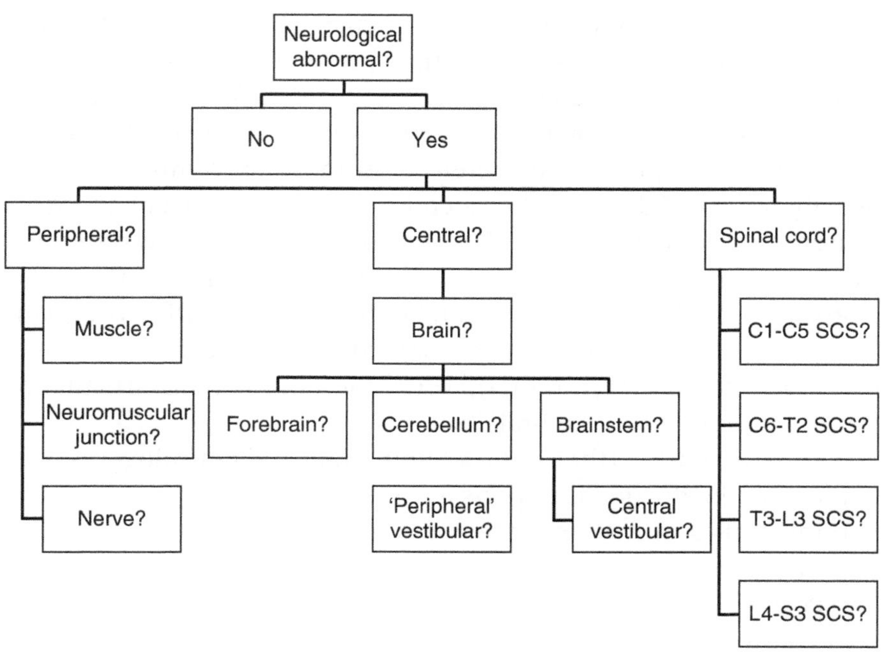

Figure 13.2 Neuroanatomical localisations (SCS=Spinal Cord Segments).

Two questions should be asked after every neurological examination:

- Is the animal neurologically normal or abnormal?
- And if abnormal where is the location of the lesion?

Once the location and distribution (focal, multi-focal or diffuse) of the lesion within the nervous or muscular system is determined (Table 13.1; Figures 13.2 and 13.3), a list of differential diagnoses can be constructed (taking into account signalment, history, pain involvement and, most importantly, the onset and progression of clinical signs). Only then, a structured plan for further investigations and treatment can be established.

The approach to the presenting complaints of weakness and collapse was discussed in detail in Chapters 6 and 7, and we therefore focus in this chapter on lesions that can present similarly to orthopaedic conditions and/or cause purely gait abnormalities. Spinal diseases can be roughly divided into two disease categories, 'myelopathic' or 'non-myelopathic'. Animals that present with back pain should be differentiated between myelopathic and non-myelopathic. Animals with concurrent neurological deficits are myelopathic, whereas those that present without neurological deficits are non-myelopathic. Which structures surrounding the spinal cord can cause pain? The nervous system's parenchyma itself has no pain receptors, and therefore, intra-parenchymal lesions are usually not painful. The only exception is neuropathic pain, which is caused by disease processes affecting the somatosensory system; for example, syringomyelia can cause neuropathic pain and the typical phantom scratching behaviour can be the only presenting complaint. Spinal diseases, which are accompanied by pain, usually affect the meninges, spinal nerve root(s), vertebrae and/or their articulations (facet joint and intervertebral disc).

Similarly to the orthopaedic examination, the neurological examination can be divided into parts as follows:

1. Hands-off examination – observation
   - Mentation and behaviour
   - Posture
   - Gait
   - Identification of abnormal involuntary movements

Table 13.1 Neuroanatomical localisations and their most common deficits.

Neuroanatomical localisation	Thoracic limbs (gait affected)	Thoracic limbs' reflexes	Pelvic limbs (gait affected)	Pelvic limbs' reflexes	Postural reactions in affected limbs	Other
C1-C5 SCS (C1-C4 vertebrae)	Yes	Intact to increased	Yes	Intact to increased	*Reduced to absent*	
C6-T2 SCS – cervical intumescence (C5-T1/2 vertebrae)	Yes	*Reduced to absent*	Yes	Intact to increased	*Reduced to absent*	
T3-L3 SCS (T2/3 – L2/3 vertebrae)	No	Intact	Yes	Intact to increased	*Reduced to absent*	Possibility of a Schiff-Sherington posture
L4-S3 SCS – lumbar intumescence	No	Intact	Yes	*Reduced to absent*	*Reduced to absent*	
Neuromuscular system – *Nerve**	Possible	*Reduced to absent*	Possible	*Reduced to absent*	*Reduced to absent*	
Neuromuscular system – *Neuromuscular Junction**	Possible	Intact (reduced)	Yes	Intact (reduced)	Intact (unless to weak)	Exercise intolerance
Neuromuscular system – *Muscle**	Possible	Intact	Possible	Intact	Intact (unless to weak)	Exercise intolerance

SCS = spinal cord segments (note: spinal cord is shorter than vertebral column). Intumescence = origin of the nerves for the specific limbs.

*see Chapter 7 for more details.

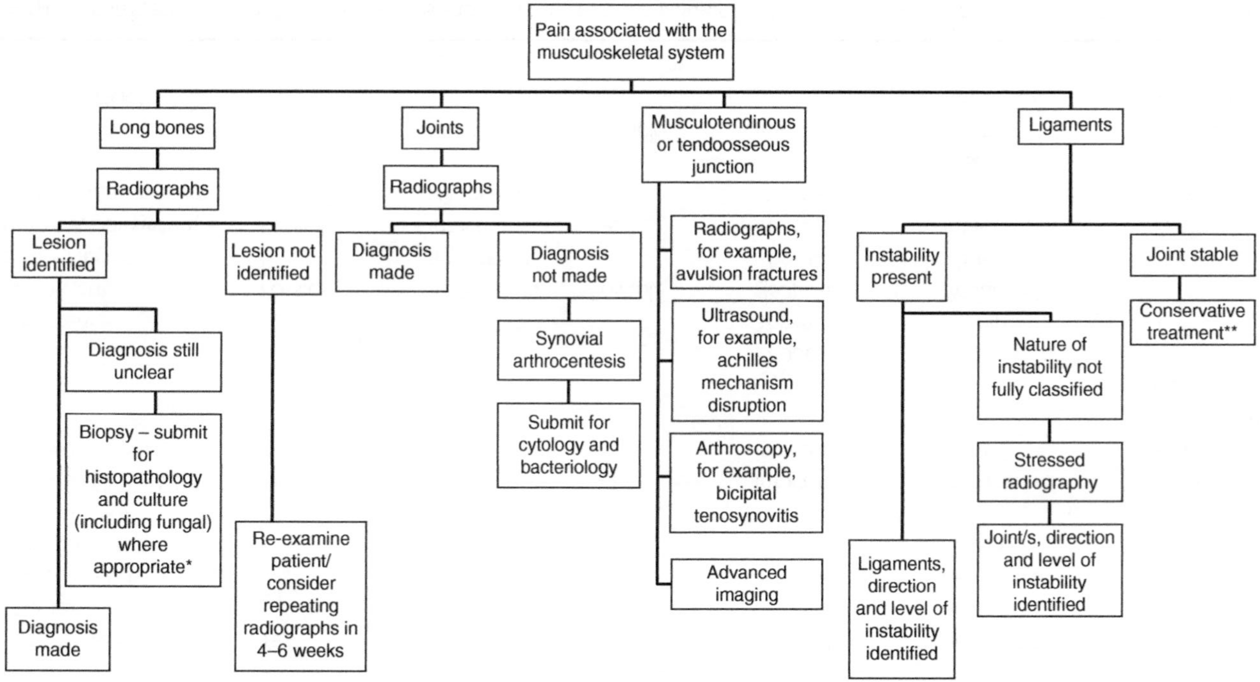

*The clinician must consider whether biopsy is indicated and the possible morbidity associated with the procedure.

** If the ligamentous injury is the result of a degenerative process it is likely to progress to joint instability.

Figure 13.3 Diagnostic work-up for the muskuloskeletal system.

2 Hands-on examination
- Postural reaction testing
- Cranial nerves assessment
- Spinal reflexes, muscle tone and size
- Sensory evaluation.

Hands-off examination – Observation

Always start with the 'big picture' (hands-off examination) and then use the hands-on examination to confirm what you have suspected to be abnormal and to help differentiate the involvement of the different parts of the neurological system. As we focus in this chapter on gait-associated spinal problems, make sure you assess at least the mentation (level and quality [behaviour changes]) and the menace response ('screening test' – this pathway tests apart from the visual system most of the other major brain compartments). If you find mentation and/or menace response deficits, a full examination is warranted.

Observe the animal from a distance, as you would do in an orthopaedic examination. Subtle neurological deficits are appreciated when the animal is walked slowly, so one would usually not examine the gait in an animal trotting unless orthopaedic disease is suspected. First of all, determine how many legs might be affected.

- Are just the pelvic limbs affected, all four limbs or just one limb?
- Which of the limbs appear to be more affected (pelvic vs. thoracic and right vs. left)?
- Does the animal have an abnormal position or curvature *(kyphosis – ∪ [ventral deviation], lordosis ∩ [dorsal deviation] or scoliosis ∫ [lateral deviation])* of the spine, which may indicate parenchymal spinal cord disease or an abnormality of the vertebral column or pain?
- *Schiff-Sherrington posture* is seen with acute thoracolumbar spinal cord lesion and is characterised by paresis or plegia of the pelvic limbs and increased tone in the thoracic limbs (high cervical lesions can also increase tone in the thoracic limbs, but unlike the Schiff-Sherington phenomenon, postural reactions will be abnormal in the thoracic limbs).

Ataxia is a lack of coordination of movement and may occur as a sensory (proprioceptive), cerebellar or vestibular ataxia (or a combination of these). *Sensory ataxia* causes a loss of sense of limb and body position, often seen as wide-based stance, swaying gait, increased (upper motor neuron – lesion localised cranial to the intumescence of the affected limbs) or decreased (lower motor neuron – lesion localised within the intumescence of the affected limbs) stride length and dragging or scuffing of the digits. It is caused by a lesion of the afferent sensory (proprioceptive) pathways in the peripheral nerves or centrally in the spinal cord, brainstem or forebrain. Sensory ataxia can be seen in dogs presented with a gait abnormality secondary to a spinal problem and needs to be differentiated from cerebellar and vestibular ataxia (Chapter 7). Sensory ataxia itself does not look necessarily different to the other type of ataxias, so to differentiate the three, one needs to take other cardinal signs into account. *Cerebellar ataxia* is characterised by an inability to control the rate and range of movement, truncal swaying, dysmetria (often hypermetria) and intention tremor. *Vestibular ataxia* is usually characterised by its cardinal signs such as head tilt, nystagmus, leaning, falling or rolling to one side.

Sensory ataxia is often associated with paresis, which is not the case for peripheral vestibular or cerebellar disease. *Paresis* is defined as a *decrease* of voluntary movement; *plegia*, on the other hand, is characterised by an *absence* of voluntary movement. Spastic (upper motor neuron) paresis or plegia occurs with disease affecting the neuronal pathways cranial to the intumescence for the limbs being affected. Flaccid paresis (lower motor neuron) occurs with disease of the motor unit (intumescence [origin of the nerves for the limb] to neuromuscular junction). Lameness can be caused not only by orthopaedic disease, but also by neurological disease (neuromuscular weakness and nerve root pain/signature).

Hands-on examination

Postural reactions test the afferent proprioceptive (sensory) and efferent motor pathways. Receptor → peripheral nerve → spinal cord → brain → spinal cord → motor unit. Subsequently, postural reactions may identify a lesion almost anywhere in the nervous system (brain, spinal cord or neuromuscular system). The gait will help to determine which limbs are affected. The postural reactions tests can help to verify which limbs are affected. They assess similar pathways, some emphasising the function of individual limbs (proprioceptive paw positioning and hopping) or groups of limbs (hemi-walking, wheel barrowing and extensor postural thrust). Patient size and temperament may not make performing every postural reaction test possible; however, completing the entire repertoire may not be necessary if a confident assessment of the patient's function can be made. Many cats do not tolerate handling of their paws, so proprioceptive (paw) positioning can be difficult to perform and interpret. Cats are invariably light enough to pick up, making the extensor postural thrust, hopping and placing (visual/tactile) useful tests. Patients should be hopped or hemi-walked away from their centre of gravity. Finding asymmetry should be considered when defining the lesion.

Spinal reflexes – gentle restraint in lateral recumbency will facilitate the testing of spinal reflexes. Changes in muscle tone should be assessed first. Stress or excitement might increase muscle tone, which may attenuate or exaggerate reflexes. Reflexes may also be attenuated due to muscle fibrosis or joint contractures or appear exaggerated if there is a lack of antagonistic muscle tone (pseudohyperreflexia seen with sciatic nerve lesion). Reflexes should therefore be interpreted only in light of the rest of the examination (gait, posture and muscle tone). A reflex should not be considered decreased or absent until multiple attempts to elicit it have been made.

- Decreased or absent reflexes are caused by a lesion in the reflex arc (receptor → peripheral nerve → spinal cord → peripheral nerve → neuromuscular junction → muscle).
- Increased reflexes result from a lack of inhibition of the reflex arc, which is caused by an alteration of the neuronal pathways cranial to the spinal segments involving the arc.
- Tendon reflexes involve percussing a tendon to cause reflex contraction of the muscle. This may be seen as movement of the limb (patellar reflex; stifle extension) or muscle contraction (biceps, triceps or gastrocnemius reflex).
- Withdrawal (flexor) reflexes are stimulated by pinching the skin between the digits and may be tested at the same time as nociception. It is important to recognise that limb withdrawal and conscious perception of pain sensation are *not* the same. The degree of flexion of individual joints should be noted.
  - Pelvic limbs assessment: focus on the hock flexion (sciatic function).
  - Thoracic limbs assessment: focus on the elbow flexion.

- The contralateral limb should be watched for evidence of a crossed-extensor reflex, which is an upper motor neuron sign.
- The perineal reflex is tested by applying a stimulus to the left and right perineum, the normal response being a bilateral contraction of the anal sphincter and flexion of the tail.
- The cutaneous-trunci reflex can be elicited by lightly plucking guard hairs along the dorsum of the spine. It is not always present in all cats.

Palpation is potentially noxious and should be performed towards the end of the examination. Extreme care must be taken if there is a history or possibility of vertebral column trauma and instability. The spine can be palpated from either end; however, if vertebral column pain is suspected from the history, it is worthwhile starting at the opposite end. Light palpation aids in detecting atrophy, swelling, masses, muscle contractures, curvatures or misalignments. The cervical spine and tail should be flexed or extended ventrally, dorsally and laterally. Symmetry of contralateral limbs should be assessed when the patient is standing. A more thorough musculoskeletal examination can be completed after spinal reflex testing while the patient is in lateral recumbency.

Nociception – assessment of nociception by nature is the most noxious part of the examination and should be left until last. A haemostat should be used, as it provides a reliably noxious stimulus. Superficial pain perception is tested by pinching a fold of skin with haemostats. Deep pain perception is tested by compressing bone (digits or tail). The stimulus should be initially gently applied and then gradually increased in intensity until a positive response is achieved, so as not to cause unnecessary pain. A positive response requires a behavioural response (vocalising, turning the head). Reflex withdrawal of the limb indicates an intact reflex arc (peripheral nerves and spinal cord segments) only, *not* conscious perception of pain requiring transmission of the stimulus up the spinal cord to the brain. The pathways that carry this sensory modality are the most resistant tracts in the spinal cord to damage; loss of deep pain perception indicates severe injury and has important prognostic implications. Cutaneous sensory testing of discrete autonomous zones or dermatomes should be performed if clinically indicated.

4 Define the lesion

Lesion localised to musculoskeletal system

Following lesion localisation, the area in question is interrogated further with the most appropriate diagnostic test (most often an imaging modality). The main diagnostic imaging tool used to assess lesions that involve the musculoskeletal system is radiography. However, the views performed and appropriate imaging modality will also be dictated by the clinician's differential diagnoses list. If long bone or joint pain is identified, then orthogonal radiographs of the affected area are recommended. If the clinician is uncertain of whether a radiographic finding may be a normal anatomic variant, radiographs of the contralateral limb may help, especially if the animal is unilaterally affected.

Careful scrutiny of the radiographs to assess whether any lesions identified are radiographically aggressive or benign should be performed. Joint effusions may be visible radiographically; for example, cruciate disease is often accompanied by cranial displacement of the infrapatellar fat pad. If there is joint instability present clinically or the cause of the pain is not apparent on the radiographs, stressed radiographs may be indicated. Stressed radiography is commonly used to identify ligamentous injuries in the distal limbs, for example, the tarsus and carpus, but it can also be used in the more proximal joints as well. Stresses can be applied in flexion, extension, valgus and varus. The joints involved and the direction of any instability will play an important role in determining the most appropriate treatment. Stressed radiography is not always required following detection of joint instability and will depend on the clinician's clinical judgement; for example, the diagnosis of cruciate disease is often inferred following detection of cranial drawer or tibial thrust in the stifle. Injuries involving the musculotendinous or tendo-osseous junction or muscles may be best imaged using ultrasound or advanced imaging techniques. Synovial arthrocentesis may help to identify inflammatory or infectious disease processes when subtle or no abnormalities are detected on survey radiographs.

Once the location of the lesion has been identified, the next step is to define the pathology of the disease process as well. The pathology of the disease process is likely to fall under one of a number of categories. The DAMNIT V scheme can be used as a helpful reminder for the different type of pathological processes that can occur (Table 13.2).

The differential list can subsequently be prioritised based on signalment, onset of clinical signs, duration, travel history, severity of clinical signs, number of limbs affected and monostotic or polyostotic bone lesions. The clinician should always question themselves whether the clinical presentation and history fit with the diagnosis. For example, an 8-year-old male Labrador presents with an acute onset of non-weight-bearing pelvic limb lameness, but has previously been diagnosed with hip dysplasia, which has been managed conservatively for many years. Why has the dog suddenly deteriorated? Hip dysplasia can present with varying degrees of lameness but rarely presents as a non-weight-bearing lameness. The clinician should consider other disease processes that may be responsible for the current clinical signs, for example, septic arthritis and intervertebral disc disease.

Lesion localised to the nervous system

Once the location of a problem within a body system is identified as the nervous system, the next key question is 'what is it?', that is, you need to define the pathology. As with orthopaedic disease, it can be helpful to remember the types of pathology that can occur on broad terms using the DAMNIT-V scheme (see details mentioned previously). However, the list of differentials for metabolic and nutritional disorders is small. The type of pathology most likely responsible for the clinical signs depends not only on the clinical course of the disease, presentation, symmetry of the deficits and pain involvement, but also on the signalment of the patient (species, breed, age, sex etc.), the geographic location of the patient and what is common in that population (Figure 13.4).

Table 13.2 Differentials to be considered for musculoskeletal disorders.

Category	Thoracic limb	Age	Pain	Onset	Patho-logical fracture	Pelvic limb	Age	Pain	Onset	Patho-logical fracture
Degenerative						Cruciate disease	Y, A	P	G, A	
						Achilles tendon rupture, for example Dobermans**	A	P	G, A	
						Plantar ligament degeneration	A	P	G	
Developmental	Elbow dysplasia	Y, A	P	G		Hip dysplasia	Y	P	G	
	Osteochondrosis dissecans	Y	P	G		Patellar luxation	Y	P	G, A	
	Retained cartilaginous core	Y		G		Osteochondrosis dissecans	Y	P	G	
	Angular limb deformities†	Y, A	P	G		Angular limb deformities†	Y, A	P	G	
Anomalous	Panosteitis	Y	P	A		Panosteitis	Y	P	A	
	Hypertrophic osteopathy	A	P	G		Hypertrophic osteopathy	A	P	G	
Metabolic	Hypertrophic osteodystrophy	Y	P	A		Hypertrophic osteodystrophy	Y	P	A	
	Renal hyperparathyroidism	A	(P)	G, A	Path	Renal hyperparathyroidism	A	(P)	G, A	Path
Neoplastic	Primary bone tumour	Y, A	P	G, A	Path	Primary bone tumour	Y, A	P	G, A	Path
	Metastatic bone tumour	A	P	G, A	Path	Metastatic bone tumour	A	P	G, A	Path

(continued overleaf)

Table 13.2 (*continued*)

Category	Thoracic limb	Age	Pain	Onset	Patho-logical fracture	Pelvic limb	Age	Pain	Onset	Patho-logical fracture
Nutritional	Nutritional hyperparathyroidism	Y	(P)	A	Path	Nutritional hyperparathyroidism	Y	(P)	A	Path
	Hypervitaminosis A	Y, A	P	G		Hypervitaminosis A	Y, A	P	G	
	Vitamin D deficiency	Y, A	(P)	G, A	Path	Vitamin D deficiency	Y, A	(P)	G, A	Path
Inflammatory/ infectious	Immune mediated polyarthritis	Y, A	P	G, A		Immune mediated polyarthritis	Y, A	P	G, A	
	Septic arthritis	Y, A	P	A		Septic arthritis	Y, A	P	A	
Traumatic	Fractures	Y, A	P	A		Fractures	Y, A	P	A	
	Luxations	Y, A	P	A		Luxations	Y, A	P	A	
	Ligamentous injuries	Y, A	P	A		Ligamentous injuries	Y, A	P	A	
	Tendon injuries	Y, A	P	A		Tendon injuries	Y, A	P	A	
	Muscle contracture†	Y, A	P	A		Muscle contracture†	Y, A	P	A	
Vascular	Bone infarct*	A		A		Bone infarct*	A		A	
						Legg Calves Perthes disease	Y	P	A, G	Path

*Bone infarcts – long-term outcome following medullary infarction is limited, but it has been associated with total hip arthroplasty and neoplasia

**An acute on chronic presentation may be appreciated with Dobermans with a degenerative achilles tendonopathy

†Condition may or may not be associated with pain

A = adult and aged dog; Y = young dog; P = can be associated with pain; Path = can cause pathological fractures; G = gradual onset; A = acute onset

(P) = pain associated with pathological fracture

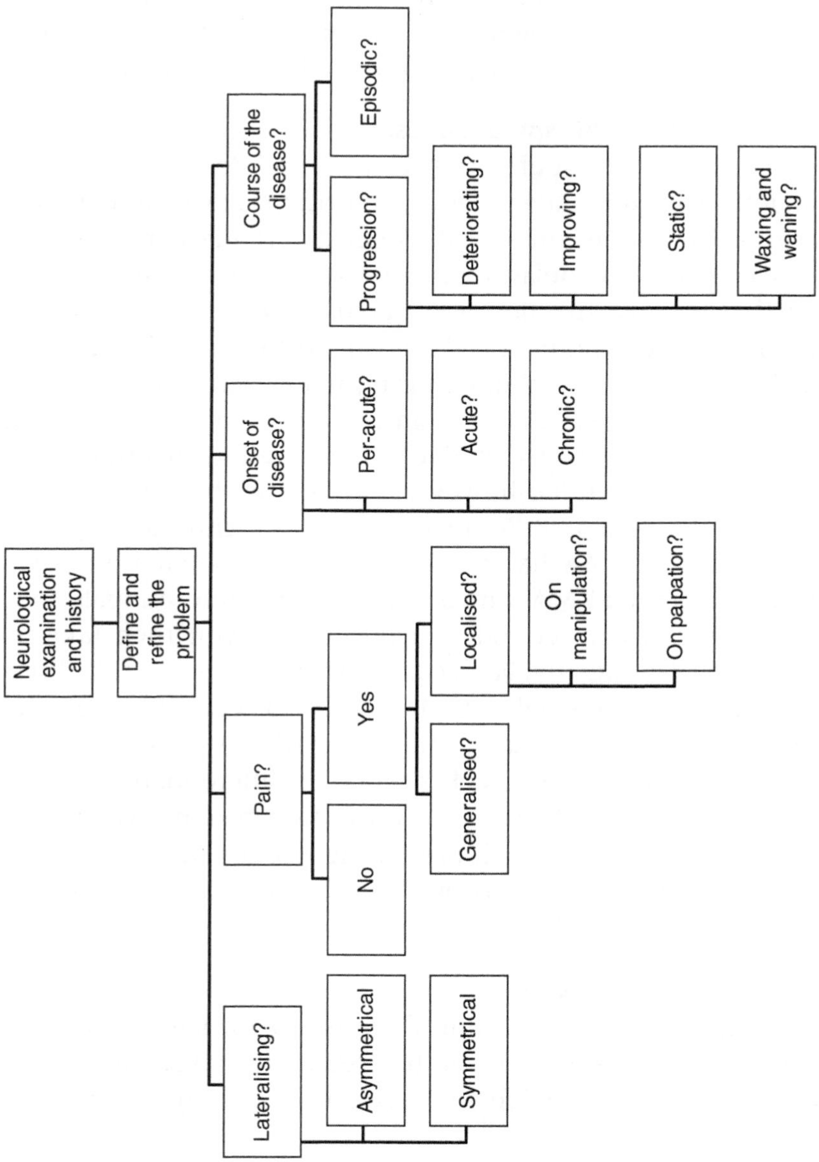

Figure 13.4 Factors to be considered for clinical reasoning in neurological conditions.

Using the five-finger ('neuro-hand-rule' [onset, clinical course, pain, lateralisation and neuroanatomical localisation – see also Chapter 7]) rule can be very helpful in clinical reasoning. After you have determined the problem by using your five-finger rule, use the signalment and see if it can help you refine it even further.

Painful non-myelopathic spinal diseases

Animals that solely present with back pain and do not show neurological deficits need to have a thorough orthopaedic examination, as polyarthritis has to be considered. Other differentials are inflammatory, infectious and neoplastic diseases. If the animal presents with a history of trauma, luxation and fractures need to be considered. As aforementioned, syringomyelia is an exception and can present as a painful condition without causing neurological deficits. As an example, syringomyelia and steroid-responsive meningitis arteritis (SRMA) can appear at first similar in presentation (painful cervical spine – non-myelopathic); however considering the clinical history, they can be differentiated. Syringomyelia has a chronic-progressive history, whereas SRMA has an acute history associated often with pyrexia. Note that SRMA can be cyclic, and some animals might have experienced pain episodes in the past. If you then take into account breed (syringomyelia occurs in small brachycephalic breeds and SRMA usually in Beagles, Border Collie, Boxers, Whippets, Jack Russell Terrier and Weimeraner) and age (SRMA usually in younger animals), you have a very high chance of differentiating the two conditions. A CSF sample can then verify the presumptive diagnosis of SRMA (depending in which part of the world you live you might need to consider infectious diseases) or an MRI scan to confirm the diagnosis of syringomyelia.

Myelopathic spinal diseases

The five-finger rule (onset, clinical course, pain, lateralisation and neuroanatomical localisation) can be used to effectively differentiate between myelopathies (Table 13.3). A couple of examples are listed as follows:

- Patients who present with peracute, non-progressive or improving, largely non-painful and lateralised neurological deficits (most often in T3-L3 spinal cord segments) have a 98% chance of having an

Table 13.3 Differentials to be considered for myelopathies.

Category	Acute non-progressive	Acute progressive	Chronic progressive
Degenerative		Type-I disc disease (P, AS, A, Y)	Cervical spondylomyelopathy (P, AS, A,Y) Type-II disk disease (P, AS, A) Degenerative myelopathy (AS, A) Demyelinating diseases (Y) Axonopathies and neuronopathies (Y) Subarachnoid diverticulum (AS, Y, A) Breed-specific myelopathies (such as Afghan hound myelopathy) (Y) Storage disease (Y)
Anomalous			Chiari-like malformation and syringomyelia (Y, A) Vertebral anomalies (Y) *Atlantoaxial (sub-)luxation (Y)* Spinal dysraphisms (Y)
Neoplastic		Primary (AS, A) Metastatic (AS, A) *Skeletal* (P, AS, A)	Nephroblastoma (AS, Y) Primary (AS, A) Metastatic (AS, A) *Skeletal* (P, AS, A)
Nutritional			*Hypervitaminosis A (Y, A)*
Inflammatory/ infectious		Distemper (P, AS, Y, A) FIP (P, AS, Y) Protozoal (P, AS, Y) MUA (P, AS, A) *Discospondylitis (P, AS, Y, A)*	Distemper (P, AS, Y, A) FIP (P, AS, Y) Protozoal (P, AS, Y) MUA (P, AS, A)

(*continued overleaf*)

Table 13.3 (*continued*)

Category	Acute non-progressive	Acute progressive	Chronic progressive
Traumatic	*Fractures (P, AS, Y, A)* Luxations (P, AS, Y, A) Contusions (AS, Y, A) ANNPE (AS, Y, A)	ANNPE (AS, Y, A)	
Vascular	Infarction (FCE; AS, Y, A) Haemmorrhage (AS, Y, A) Vascular malformations (AS, Y)		

(A = adult and aged dog; Y = young dog; P = can be associated with pain; AS = can be asymmetrical in presentation [one side more affected than the other]; MUA = meningomyelitis of unknown aetiology); ANNPE = acute noncompressive nucleus pulposus extrusion. Diseases that can also present with spinal pain without causing neurological signs are in italics.

ischaemic myelopathy such as fibrocartilaginous embolism (FCE) or high velocity but low volume disc prolapse (acute noncompressive nucleus pulposus extrusion [ANNPE]).

- Hansen type-I disc disease (intervertebral disc extrusion) is best characterised as an acute onset, deteriorating, painful and occasionally lateralised myelopathy (often at T3-L3 spinal cord segments). Ninety percent of patients presenting with these clinical signs will have Hansen type-I disease.
- In contrast, Hansen type-II (intervertebral disc protrusion) has a more chronic onset, is often stable, but still painful.
- Meningo(encephalo)myelitis of unknown aetiology (MUA) can present with an acute onset, deteriorating painful myelopathy. MUA is four times more likely to present as a multifocal neuroanatomical localisation (multiple spinal cord segments and/or brain). Many of the animals will also have mentation changes and cranial nerve deficits.

These examples demonstrate that thinking pathophysiologically and using the five-finger rule can refine the differential list significantly. If you then also take demographics and signalment into account, you have a very high chance of identifying the most likely diagnosis before embarking on diagnostics. Many of the neurological conditions will require advanced imaging and/or CSF analysis, but funds are limited, and the aforementioned approach can provide you with the framework to narrow down diagnostics to the most essential or provide the owner with a presumptive diagnosis.

Conclusion

The patient presenting with a gait abnormality may have orthopaedic disease, neurological disease or both. The orthopaedic and neurological examinations are the key diagnostic tools that will enable the clinician to formulate a rational differential list and plan appropriate diagnostic procedures to confirm the diagnosis.

CHAPTER 14

Pruritus and scaling

Andrea V. Volk & Jill E. Maddison
The Royal Veterinary College, Department of Clinical Science and Services, London, UK

Introduction

Pruritus and scaling are two of the most common skin complaints in companion animals, particularly dogs. There are many causes of these clinical signs, and the purpose of this chapter is not to discuss the details of specific skin diseases, but to give some background to the pathogenesis of pruritus and scaling and provide a structured approach to the assessment of the patient with pruritus and/or scaling.

Pruritus

Pruritus is an unpleasant sensation of the skin provoking the urge to scratch. The physiological rationale for pruritus is to eliminate parasites. Pruritus is an autonomous, pain-independent sensation, which is transmitted to the thalamus via itch-specific neuronal pathways. Recognition of pruritus leads to scratching, which induces pain to override the itch sensation. Pruritus-related projections to the thalamus are actively inhibited by pain-processing neurons and vice versa. Once these pain neurons are suppressed, the itch sensation may increase. An example is seen in humans receiving morphine treatment. We need to remember that in animals, we are only able to observe scratching, which we interpret as a behavioural response to itch.

Clinical Reasoning in Small Animal Practice, First Edition.
Jill E. Maddison, Holger A. Volk and David B. Church.

Pathophysiology of pruritus

An understanding of the pathophysiology of pruritus improves the clinician's appreciation of the rationale for anti-pruritic management strategies.

Pruriceptors

Pruriceptors are specific free nerve endings in the epidermis, dermoepidermal junction and dermis. After stimulation via mediators (see the following section), the pruritic sensation is transmitted via afferent fibres, slow conducting C-fibres to the dorsal horn of the spinal cord and via central itch-specific neuronal pathways to the thalamus.

Pruritic mediators

The cytokine IL-31 has been identified as the major pruritic cytokine in people and canines, predominantly produced by T_H2 cells. Other mediators stimulating pruriceptors are IL-2 (IL-6, IL-8 presumed), predominantly from T cells and mast cells, neuropeptides from keratinocytes, kinins (including bradykinin), amines (including histamine), proteases (produced by e.g. neutrophils, bacteria, fungal organism, mast cells and other inflammatory cells), prostaglandins, leukotrienes, neurophins and substance P. Interestingly, not every mediator induces in every species or even every dog breed itch or even the same level of itch; the specific mechanisms to explain these differences in detail are still to be elucidated.

The presence of pruritic mediators in cutaneous inflammation will lead to a vicious cycle of perpetuating itch and inflammation. Chronic stimulation of keratinocytes, Merkel cells, mast cells and Langerhans cells has been shown to produce nerve growth factor (NGF). This leads to an increasing number of itch fibres in the epidermis and dermis. This is one of the likely underlying mechanisms that explains the increasing difficulties that can occur in controlling chronic itch, particularly when appropriate therapy has not been started in an earlier phase.

Central factors

The itch threshold in humans has been shown to be reduced in the following circumstances:

- at night
- by increased skin temperatures

- by decreased skin hydration
- with increased psychic stress.

Stressful situations may potentiate pruritus through the release of various opioid peptides. Competing cutaneous sensations (pain, touch, heat and cold) can magnify or reduce the sensation of pruritus. Thus, the sensation of pruritus is often increased at night, as other sensory input is low.

Anti-pruritics

Glucocorticoids continue to be the mainstay of a first-line anti-pruritic therapy and are consistently efficacious in the majority of cases. However, ciclosporin and the new narrow spectrum anti-pruritic drug, oclaticinib, are very useful alternatives to glucocorticoids and are reported to have similar efficacy. In addition, a variety of non-steroidal therapies for the management of pruritus have been explored, although they have very variable efficacy and there is little evidence to support their use. These include maropitant (anti-substance P), cannabinoids, kappa opioid receptor agonists, agonists for the cold and menthol receptor TRPM 8 (transient receptor potential subfamily M member 8).

Diagnostic approach to the pruritic patient

1 Define the problem

Owners may not always recognise that their pet's behaviour is occurring because they are pruritic. It is, therefore, important to make owners aware of signs of itch other than obvious scratching, such as:

- rolling
- rubbing
- chewing
- scooting
- head shaking
- licking.

There is a validated visual analogue scale of pruritus available to objectify owners' subjective perception of pruritus, and this can also be useful in monitoring the effect of treatment on the level of itch. It can be helpful to enquire whether, if there is a low level of pruritus, the owner feels the animal has a good quality of life despite the itch, as, for example, allergic patients will never be itch-free.

These discussions will aid in putting the owners' expectations in a realistic light, which is very important for the management of chronic pruritic cases.

2 Define the system

In pruritus, the skin is the primary system affected. The initiating cause may originate from within the skin (primary skin disease) or be secondarily affected due to systemic disorders (such as biliary and renal disorders), neuropathic (Chapter 13) or compulsive behaviour disorders (Chapter 7).

3 Define the location

Distribution

The distribution of pruritus is a very important guide for the differential diagnoses list. In ectoparasitic diseases such as scabies pruritus is seen predominantly on lesser haired areas such as pinnal margins and extensor areas of elbow and tarsus; demodicosis is mostly found in a facial and pedal distribution; fleas and *Cheyletiella* commonly cause pruritus primarily on the dorsal rump. In contrast, allergic dogs and cats predominantly have pruritus on the flexural areas and medioventral aspects of the body, respectively.

4 Define the lesion

Major causes

Many skin diseases will cause pruritus, but the major ones are (Figure 14.1) as follows:

- Ectoparasites (and endoparasites)
- Infection (bacterial, fungal, viral and protozoal)
- Allergic skin disease (flea-, food-, environmental hypersensitivities).

Rate of onset

A rapid onset of pruritus is most often associated with acute secondary superficial pyoderma, *Malassezia* dermatitis, ectoparasite infestation, particularly *Sarcoptes*, *Cheyletiella* or fleas or ingestion of an ingredient to which the patient is hypersensitive. In patients with environmental

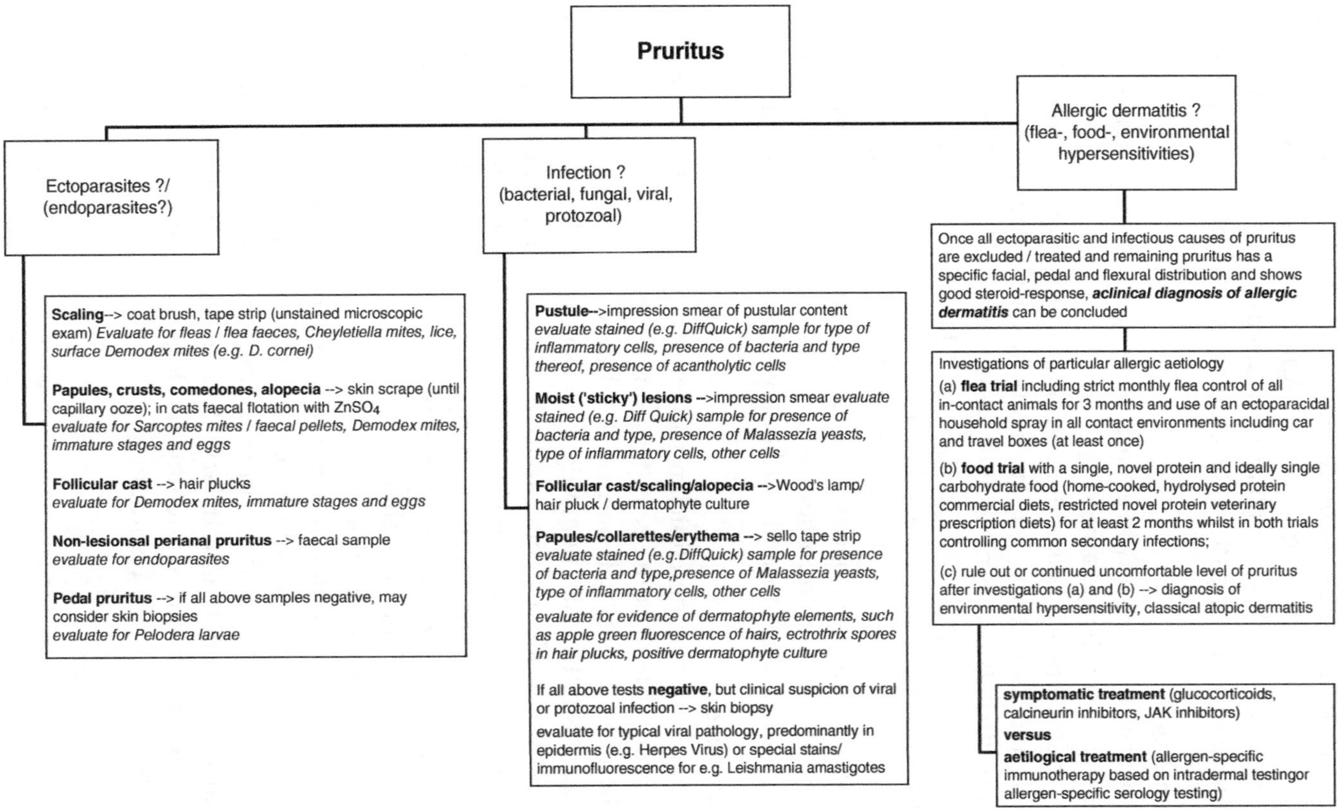

Figure 14.1 Flow diagram to the diagnostic approach of pruritus in companion animals.

hypersensitivities, there is more likely a gradual increase in pruritus when entering their allergy season. Another cause of acute pruritus can be the onset of a complete new disease process, for example a chronic mildly atopic patient developing epitheliotropic lymphoma.

Seasonality

If the pruritus recurs only in a particular season, it may suggest a likely triggering factor. For example:

- Flea-related pruritus is more common in the summer months
- Grass hypersensitivity is more likely in spring and summer months
- House dust-/storage mite hypersensitivity is more likely to show pronounced flares from October until January/February.

Perennial itch could be related to food hypersensitivity and/or house dust-/storage mite hypersensitivity. In addition, itch can increase due to psychogenic causes as a result of certain activities within the home environment (e.g. stress of visitors, building works, moving home, new animals and beloved owners in hospital).

Primary lesions

It is important for the clinician to identify primary skin lesions and differentiate them from secondary ones. For example, the presence of follicular pustules will narrow the differential list (pyoderma, pustular dermatophytosis; pemphigus foliaceus, further sterile pustular diseases) and guide the clinician to the correct diagnostic test (impression smear of pustular content) to either confirm the diagnosis or lead to the next diagnostic test. In comparison, identification of papules would lead to the consideration of scabies, other ectoparasites, early pyoderma (if follicular) or allergic dermatitis. Skin scrapings would be the appropriate test in these cases.

Should the skin look completely normal, but the animal is pruritic, allergic skin disease should be considered (pruritus *sine materia, i.e. clinically normal apart from pruritus*) as well as systemic disorders (in particular renal and biliary disorders), neuropathic disorders (head/neck phantom scratching in dogs with syringomyelia) and compulsive behaviour disorders.

Secondary lesions

Secondary lesions, such as excoriations, lichenifications, scars, fissures, callus and necrosis may not be very helpful in leading to a diagnosis. They can, however, indicate to the clinician the level of pruritus and chronicity of the disease. Other secondary lesions such as collarettes, erosions and ulcers may have some diagnostic value and may be the only lesion observed when the primary lesion is fragile such as vesicles or pustules in autoimmune diseases.

Secondary infections

Secondary infections of the skin are a frequent complication of many pruritic disorders and will be in themselves pruritic. Thus, once infection has been identified that needs antimicrobial treatment, it is best to avoid glucocorticoids in the first instance. Pruritus and skin lesions will be re-assessed upon resolution of the infectious process and will then provide further clues as to the aetiology of the pruritus. However, a subset of allergic dogs presents with recurrent pyoderma as the only clinical sign and may be itch-free once the pyoderma has been treated and in between episodes.

Self-trauma

Unfortunately, self-trauma subsequent to pruritus will result in the release of more mediators of pruritus. Thus, a vicious itch–scratch cycle is initiated, although the original inciting cause may have resolved. Increased numbers of itch fibres will further enhance pruritus, and hyperaesthesia of the skin will develop over time.

Scaling

Most scaling disorders in human medicine are associated with increased and changed sebum production, hence the clinical descriptive term seborrhoea. Seborrhoea used in the veterinary context is a misnoma. Seborrhoea translates into 'flow of grease'. In the veterinary patient, dry (previously termed 'seborrhea sicca') and greasy ('seborrhea oleosa') *keratinisation disorders* are recognised equally. As a result, in the last two decades, the nomenclature has been changed to keratinisation/cornification disorder, an aetiological term.

The terms keratinisation and cornification are often used interchangeably, although strictly speaking, keratinisation is only a part of the cornification process. Keratinisation is the differentiation and aggregation of intermediate filaments within the keratinocyte.

Further processes involved in cornification are formation of the lipid and cornified envelope (cross-linking of proteins), dissolution of nucleus and all cell organelles and desquamation.

Diagnostic approach to scaling

1 Define the problem

The clinical presentation of a patient (Figure 14.2) with a keratinisation disorder will include increased scaling and in addition may include the following:

- greasiness and/or malodour of the coat,
- further coat, claw or foot pad changes such as
  - dull, brittle hair or claws
  - thickening with or without fissures on the foot pads.

2 Define the system

In keratinisation disorders, the skin is the primary system. However, the underlying trigger may not originate from the skin but be an endocrinopathy (e.g. hypothyroidism, hyperadrenocorticism and sex hormone imbalances), nutritional or systemic neoplasia. Thus, when a keratinisation disorder is observed, it is very important to determine whether it is a primary (i.e. idiopathic/genetic) or secondary (metabolic, nutritional and neoplastic) disorder. In secondary disorders, if the cause has been identified and if successful treatment is possible, the keratinisation disorder may be cured. However, primary keratinisation disorders are usually not curable, and life-long management will likely be necessary to achieve an acceptable quality of life for the patient and owner.

Important clues

Primary keratinisation disorders manifest more commonly in young animals, either as focal or as generalised process. Certain breeds have been recognised to be more likely affected. A primary disease is also more likely in an otherwise healthy animal, and not only skin, but also coat, claws and footpads are affected in generalised disorders.

Secondary keratinisation disorders should be suspected if the clinician is presented with a middle-aged to older animal with either first

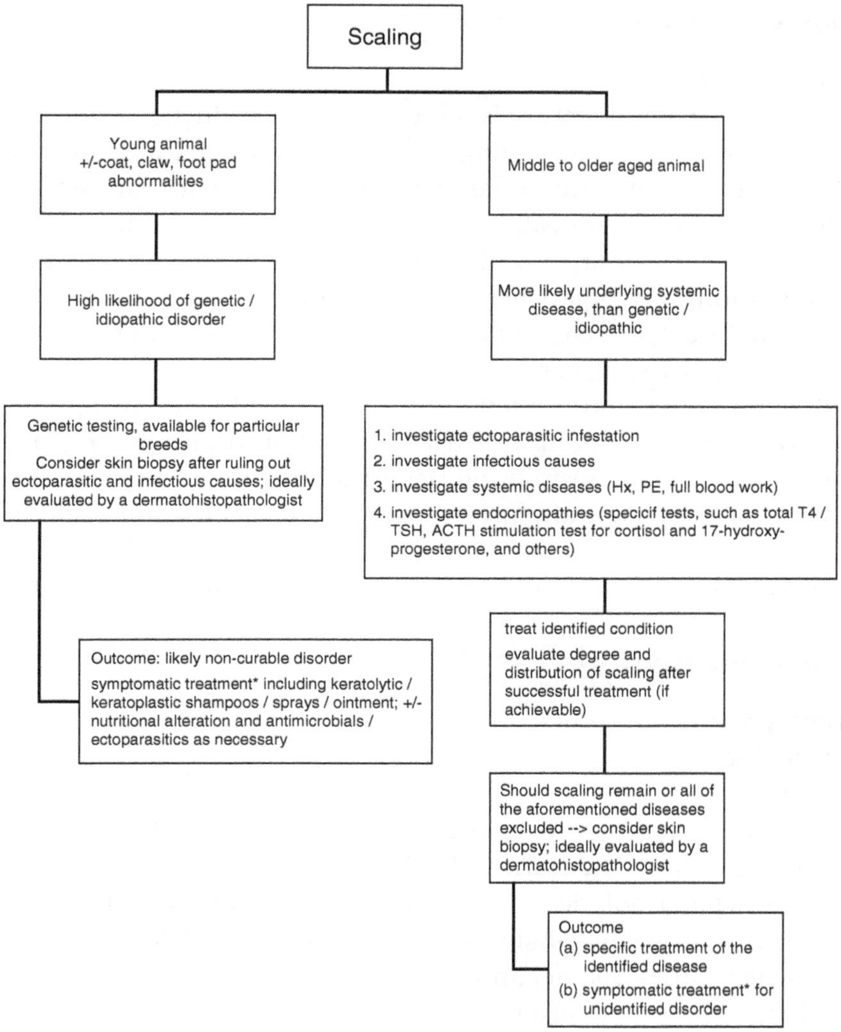

Figure 14.2 Flow diagram to the diagnostic approach of scaling presentation in companion animals (Hx = history; PE = physical examination).

time skin complaint or scaling as a new presentation. An underlying cause must be investigated. As the patient is of middle to older age, full physical examination and history taken including any preceding drug exposure is imperative. In these cases, the presence or absence of pruritus will help narrow down the differential list.

3 Define the location

Classification

Clinically, the main feature is increased scale production, which may be associated with thickening (lichenification) of the skin, excess grease production and inflammation with or without secondary infection (bacterial/fungal). The visible scales derive from the *stratum corneum*, the upper layer of the epidermis. They are either just a cell shell without any organelles (orthokeratotic corneocyte) or contain a retained nucleus (parakeratotic corneocyte). The latter type often clinically appears thicker.

Examples of keratinisation disorders include the following:

- Focal genetically predisposed keratinisation disorder (dry) in the ear margin dermatosis in the Dachshund
- Generalised genetically predisposed oily keratinisation disorder in Bassett Hounds
- Acquired keratinisation disorders as seen in hypothyroid dogs.

4 Define the lesion

Primary scaling disorders

Generalised

- Ichthyosis
  - Epidermolytic (with epidermal loosening towards vesicle/bulla formation) in the Norfolk Terrier
  - Non-epidermolytic (without epidermal loosening and epidermal retention) in the Golden Retriever, Jack Russell Terrier, Cavalier King Charles Spaniel and other breeds
- Altered zinc metabolism
  - Zinc-responsive dermatosis syndrome I in Nordic dog breeds
  - Lethal acrodermatitis in the English Bullterrier.

Focal

- Ear margin dermatosis in Dachshunds
- Nasal parakeratosis in Labradors
- Nasodigital hyperkeratosis in Dogues de Bordeaux, Irish Terrier and Labradors
- Idiopathic facial dermatosis in the Persian cat

- Stud tail, most prevalent in longhaired cats
- Feline chin acne.

Secondary scaling disorders

Focal or generalised depending on the cause

- Ectoparasites – in particular
  - *Cheyletiella*
  - *Sarcoptes*
  - fleas
  - *Demodex*
- Infection
  - pyoderma
  - dermatophytosis
  - leishmaniasis
  - FeLV
  - associated giant cell dermatosis
- Endocrinopathies – for example
  - hypothyroididsm
  - hyperadrenocorticism
  - sex hormone imbalances
- Autoimmune diseases – for example
  - sebaceous adenitis
  - lupus erythematosus
  - pemphigus foliaceus
  - erythema multiforme
- Cutaneous adverse drug reactions
- Neoplastic
  - primary cutaneous neoplasm
    - for example epitheliotropic T-cell lymphoma
  - cutaneous paraneoplastic syndrome
    - for example secondary to thymoma
- Nutrition
  - zinc-responsive dermatosis syndrome II in large breed dogs with a zinc-deficient or phytate-rich diet
  - Vitamin A deficiency
- Metabolic
  - superficial necrolytic dermatitis ('hepatocutaneous syndrome').

Diagnostics

Diagnostic tools for the assessment of the patient with scaling include those that assess local cutaneous disorders such as ectoparasites and infection (skin scrapes, cytology and culture) and those that assess systemic causes of keratinisation disorders. The presence of pruritus is a clue that may guide the choice of tests, although the absence of pruritus does not rule out local disorders. For example, most ectoparasitic infestations are pruritic; however, demodicosis can be non-pruritic. Most infectious processes within the skin are pruritic; however, dermatophytosis and leishmaniasis can be non-pruritic. Note that an underlying endocrinopathy such as hyperadrenocorticism may alter the sensation of an otherwise pruritic disorder.

Thus, if the patient is non-pruritic and/or has other clinical signs suggestive of a systemic disorder, haematology and biochemistry should be evaluated; total thyroxine levels and TSH should be measured while keeping in mind the possibility of sick euthyroid syndrome. If hyperadrenocorticism is a feasible diagnosis when the signalment of the patient is considered (e.g. middle aged to older dogs or cats with uncontrolled diabetes mellitus), a urine cortisol:creatinine ratio can be measured. The urine sample must be collected at home in a stress-free environment. If negative, this rules out hyperadrenocorticism; if positive, provocative testing of the adrenal gland such as ACTH stimulation test or low dose dexamethasone suppression test is needed. To investigate potential sexual hormone imbalances, evaluating 17-hydroxy-progesterone levels in an ACTH stimulation test would be useful.

Skin biopsy

Once ectoparasitic, infectious and systemic causes of scaling such as endocrinopathies have been ruled out, skin biopsies may be useful. Skin biopsies should be taken from the affected skin, including all three layers (epidermis, dermis and subcutis) without prior manipulation of the skin (no cleaning, no scrubbing and no antiseptics) and as 'large' as possible depending on the body site (ideally 8 mm diameter). Interpreting the histopathology of skin biopsies is not easy – it requires time (usually triple the time of any other organ sample to read) and special interest of the pathologist, particularly in scaling disorders. Thus, ideally, the biopsies should be sent to a dermatohistopathologist, who might also be interested in seeing clinical pictures of the case and having a detailed discussion with the clinician once the histopathology has been described.

Care should be taken *not* to biopsy scaling disorders in the first instance, as if infection and/or ectoparasite infestation is/are present, the histopathology will only reflect that, although there might be an underlying sebaceous adenitis. In addition, owners should always be prepared that histopathology is not a 'for definite–diagnosing' test; it may well be non-diagnostic. In cases where the biopsy seems non-diagnostic, the histopathology could be reviewed by another pathologist/dermatologist or the effect of a trial treatment could be evaluated, depending on the clinician's strongest clinical suspicion.

In conclusion

Pruritus and scaling are common clinical signs in animals, which reflect a myriad of causes. The keys to reaching a rational differential list and confirming the diagnosis where possible lie in careful examination of the patient to document the specific type and distribution of lesions, the recognition of primary and secondary skin lesions and appreciation that both pruritus and scaling can be due to systemic disease and not just local disease.

Index

Note: Page numbers in *italics* represent figures, those in **bold** represent tables

Clinical Reasoning in Small Animal Practice, First Edition.
Jill E. Maddison, Holger A. Volk and David B. Church.